AGING, BIOTECHNOLOGY, AND THE FUTURE

AGING, BIOTECHNOLOGY, AND THE FUTURE

Edited by

CATHERINE Y. READ, PH.D., R.N.
Associate Professor of Adult Health
Boston College Connell School of Nursing
Chestnut Hill, Massachusetts

ROBERT C. GREEN, M.D., M.P.H.
Professor of Neurology, Genetics, and Epidemiology and
Co-Director, Alzheimer's Disease
Clinical and Research Program
Boston University Schools of Medicine and Public Health
Boston, Massachusetts

MICHAEL A. SMYER, PH.D.
Professor and Director
Center on Aging and Work
Boston College
Chestnut Hill, Massachusetts

The Johns Hopkins University Press
Baltimore

© 2008 The Johns Hopkins University Press
All rights reserved. Published 2008
Printed in the United States of America on acid-free paper
9 8 7 6 5 4 3 2 1

The Johns Hopkins University Press
2715 North Charles Street
Baltimore, Maryland 21218-4363
www.press.jhu.edu

Library of Congress Cataloging-in-Publication Data

Aging, biotechnology, and the future / edited by Catherine Y. Read,
Robert C. Green, and Michael A. Smyer.
       p. ; cm.
    Includes bibliographical references and index.
    ISBN-13: 978-0-8018-8788-8 (hardcover : alk. paper)
    ISBN-10: 0-8018-8788-7 (hardcover : alk. paper)
    1. Aging—Genetic aspects. 2. Longevity—Genetic aspects.
3. Alzheimer's disease—Diagnosis. 4. Alzheimer's disease—Genetic
aspects. 5. Medical genetics—Social aspects. 6. Genetic engineering—
Moral and ethical aspects. 7. Centenarians. I. Read, Catherine Y.
II. Green, Robert C., 1954– III. Smyer, Michael A.
    [DNLM: 1. Aging—genetics. 2. Aging—psychology. 3. Alzheimer
Disease—genetics. 4. Genetic Techniques—trends. 5. Health Services for
the Aged. 6. Population Dynamics. WT 104 A2674043 2008]
    QP86.A35927 2008
    612.6'7—dc22

                                                      2007036860

A catalog record for this book is available from the British Library.

*Special discounts are available for bulk purchases of this book. For
more information, please contact Special Sales at 410-516-6936 or
specialsales@press.jhu.edu.*

The Johns Hopkins University Press uses environmentally friendly book
materials, including recycled text paper that is composed of at least 30
percent post-consumer waste, whenever possible. All of our book papers
are acid-free, and our jackets and covers are printed on paper with
recycled content.

To our families . . . past, present, and future

CONTENTS

PREFACE

Two revolutions will affect the well-being of older Americans in the twenty-first century: the demographic revolution of an aging society and the scientific revolution of molecular biology. This book focuses on the effects of advances in biotechnology on an aging population. These effects cannot be described by any one author or from any one disciplinary perspective or for any one subset of the population. Humans are a diverse species with individual goals, values, and resources. Ethical issues arise at the intersection of biotechnological advances, demographic change, and personal priorities.

Recent advances in biotechnology and our newfound understanding of the human genome have opened a door to exciting new possibilities for improving the quality and duration of life, albeit with many caveats. The idea of replacing ailing organs or tissues with healthy ones created from stem cells is gaining widespread acceptance, yet the use of related technology to reproduce an entire human being generally evokes condemnation. Using a genetic test to determine whether a person is at increased risk for colon cancer seems prudent because early colonoscopy can target a malignancy for removal before it becomes lethal, but genetic testing for incurable diseases such as Huntington or Alzheimer disease may have psychosocial consequences that outweigh any potential benefit. Antiaging technologies have a tremendous marketing appeal, but there are significant limitations to their benefits and a lack of regulatory control on their use.

In an effort to further the dialogue on these difficult topics, we gathered nationally known scholars from the fields of medicine, law, biology, psychology, gerontology, nursing, philosophy, ethics, and religion in Boston in March 2005. The National Institute on Aging and the Jesuit Institute of Boston College provided funding for this unique interdisciplinary forum, with the goals of stimulating critical thinking and new ideas about the ongoing revolution in genetics and biotechnology, encouraging collaborative linkages among scientists from different disciplines, and addressing the multiple related ethical and social dilemmas. We sought to find out more about the technologies that will affect lifespan or the concerns of aging, gather data about the shift in the age of the world's population, and talk about the characteristics of the "oldest old."

Most of all, we wanted to learn what the experts from diverse disciplines would say about the societal effects of an aging population and the significance of biotechnology. This volume is a compilation of chapters by these experts, and it includes descriptions of original research, discussions of philosophical perspectives on the topics, and responses to the ideas presented at the forum. Each chapter represents a unique and often provocative perspective on the effect of the biotechnology revolution on an aging society. Predictions about the future are tentative at best, and the discussions generally raise more questions than they answer. The challenge will be to unify the perspectives of multiple disciplines and cope with change in a manner that is beneficial to all.

If you take a group of 6-year-olds and a group of 66-year-olds, which will be more diverse? The 66-year-olds. Why? A combination of genetic predispositions, lifestyle, and life experiences make humans more different from each other as they age. In the twenty-first century those differences may also be affected by the tools of biotechnology, and this possibility raises important issues. The French philosopher Michel Philibert (1979) posed three questions that form the basis of our interdisciplinary conversation on aging, biotechnology, and the future: Of aging, what can we know? About aging, what must we hope? With aging, what can we do? This book follows Philibert's lead by asking these questions as a way to introduce the areas of inquiry needed to engage ethical issues for an aging society in an era of biotechnology.

Richard Sprott (chap. 1) opens the discussion of the first question—Of aging, what can we know?—with data about the expanding human life expectancy and the resultant shift in the age of the population. By 2030 the number of people in the United States aged 65 and older is expected to double (National Center for Health Statistics, 2005). This shift will result in certain social and economic burdens, but Sprott is optimistic that these will be offset by the development of effective new therapies for age-related diseases. He says that we are "in the midst of the most exciting and important scientific era in the history of the world." The recent unraveling of the human genome opens up intriguing possibilities, such as the ability to design drugs based on an individual's genetic makeup and the potential to replace defective genes or gene products. Sprott is particularly enthusiastic about the application of knowledge about telomeres. Telomeres are stretches of DNA that protect the ends of chromosomes, much as a plastic tip on a shoelace prevents fraying of the lace. An enzyme called telomerase adds DNA fragments to the ends of the telomeres during replication, but its function diminishes after many cell replications, and the telomeres shorten until they can no longer divide. Theoretically, then, addition of telomerase to healthy cells could keep them from aging, and removal of telomerase from cancer cells could prevent their uncontrolled growth.

The promise of harnessing scientific concepts for antiaging technology must be viewed in the context of its ethical and socially responsible use. Real improvements in what Sprott calls the "healthspan" are likely to become available, but with them will come commercialization, media hype, confusion, and controversy. The complexity of genetics and biotechnology renders consumers susceptible to hucksters, and the antiaging industry preys on those who believe a charlatan's claim that the key to a long life may be found in a bottle of pills or a visit to a spa. Sprott is most concerned about the dilemma of resource allocation in relation to antiaging technologies. This concern is echoed in Fernando Guerra's commentary in chapter 2 about ensuring equitable distribution of life-extending products and services in a diverse aging society. Guerra urges the health care community to participate actively in the policy arena and cautions against the development of expensive new treatments and interventions that are not available to persons with limited financial resources.

In Part II we turn to another of Philibert's questions: About aging, what must we hope? Recent speculations in the scholarly and popular literatures have focused on the quest for immortality. Through cloning, stem cell techniques, and other approaches, the indefinite extension of life seems almost feasible. At the same time, important ethical issues arise with this potential goal. Apart from the scientific plausibility of such a future, a more fundamental question arises: Are there ethical qualms regarding such a goal? And if so, what are they and what is their basis?

In chapter 3 George Annas opens the discussion about lifespan extension by exploring it from the perspective of the human species and human rights.

Proponents of technologies for extreme inheritable genetic modifications or human cloning would be participating in species endangering activities that Annas likens to the use of nuclear weapons. Such activities threaten the essence of humanity itself by directing evolution toward what has been termed the "posthuman." Thomas Shannon elaborates on the concept of the posthuman (or "transhuman") in chapter 4. The transhumanist viewpoint is based on the premise that humans are currently only in the early phase of their development as a species. Whereas our evolution from prehuman to human was shaped primarily by natural selection in the context of environmental factors like climate and food supply, our ongoing evolution from human to posthuman is shaped also by the process of culture. Cultural factors impose goals, desires, and values on evolution and may attempt to override biology and natural selection. One inevitable result of this phenomenon is a quest for life extension and genetic enhancement, and the transhumanists carry this to an extreme with various prescriptions for transcending the causes of mortality and attaining ageless perfection. Both Annas and Shannon agree that such narrowly self-centered extremism ignores the common good of the species. Annas warns that this approach can be characterized by a slippery slope into neoeugenics, and he proposes wording for a document that would impose a worldwide ban on all efforts to initiate a pregnancy using intentionally modified genetic material or reproductive cloning technology.

Extremism aside, biotechnology has potential for mitigating the effects of the degenerative diseases that affect millions of older adults. In chapter 5 Robert Lanza reports on recent advances in somatic cell nuclear transfer (SCNT). In SCNT, a cell can be cloned, or copied, by having its DNA inserted into an egg with the nucleus removed. This reconstructed egg cell can be implanted in a uterus and stimulated to develop into a new animal, a process called reproductive cloning. Scientists generally agree that reproductive cloning is inappropriate in humans. However, these reconstructed eggs can also be cultured in a lab to produce additional stem cells or coaxed into forming specific tissues for medical use (therapeutic cloning). These cells and tissues can be engineered to produce missing proteins or perform the functions of diseased organs. For example, persons with Parkinsonism, who have debilitating motor symptoms as a result of a deficiency of dopamine in the basal ganglia of the brain, could theoretically have their functional capacity restored with the implantation of cloned dopamine-producing neurons. For persons with type 1 diabetes, whose pancreatic β-islet cells have been destroyed by an immune reaction, SCNT may be able to provide insulin-producing replacement β-islet cells. Because these tissues are grown from the patient's own stem cells, the risk of rejection is nearly eliminated. In addition to these therapeutic benefits for specific diseases, Lanza's studies have demonstrated that it is possible to take a senescent cell and restore it to a youthful state with lengthened telomeres and a restored lifespan (Lanza et al., 2000).

These insights from basic science support Sprott's premise that antiaging technologies are on the horizon, and this leads to several dilemmas that Maxwell Mehlman examines in chapter 6. Should the goal of these technologies be freedom from chronic disease, decelerated aging, or a prolonged human lifespan? Mehlman argues against projects that aim to prolong life merely for life's sake. Should antiaging technologies be regarded as therapies or enhancements? The answer to that question depends, in part, on one's attitude toward natural aging and has implications for how such technologies will be paid for and whether they are determined to be legal. Finally, Mehlman tackles the question of how antiaging technologies should be regulated. Oversight of medical practice is the responsibility of individual states, and there are numerous gaps and weaknesses in the system, especially with regard to antiaging and alternative medicine products (U.S. General Accounting Office, 2001). Dietary supplements, cosmetic medicine, and off-label uses of prescription drugs pose challenges to regulatory agencies. Mehlman concludes that strict regulation of the antiaging industry is absolutely essential to protect consumer safety, prevent adverse economic consequences, and ensure equitable access to technologies.

In chapter 7 Karen Lebacqz expands the discussion of equitable access to antiaging technologies by framing it as a question of justice. She warns against technology that would extend the normal lifespan or change our sense of what a normal lifespan should be, but she supports interventions that cure diseases like diabetes or restore lost physiological functions. Access to such interventions is likely to be most available to the rich, the insured, the literate, persons in developed nations, and others of privilege. Lebacqz argues that what we must ultimately hope for about aging should be based on a consensus about the meaning and purpose of human life and a commitment to equitable distribution.

Philibert's final question—What we can do with aging?—is addressed in parts III and IV. On the continuum of desirable and undesirable options related to aging, healthy centenarians represent one extreme, and persons with Alzheimer disease represent the other. The answer to the question about what we can do with aging may be found, in part, by studying centenarians, a group of individuals who have successfully prolonged their lifespan without the use of modern biotechnology. Centenarians are the scouts at the frontier of aging who bring back reports of what a very long life might be like and draw attention to interesting scientific and ethical issues. What are the individual and social factors that contribute to becoming a centenarian? What role can and does genetics play in reaching this milestone? When does it become an individual or societal milestone? But we also have much to learn from patients and families challenged by Alzheimer disease, a prototype for the study of genetic testing for disordered aging. Do people want to know their probability of developing a debilitating condition? Can predictive genetic testing be safely, ethically, sensitively, and equitably offered? Will such information alter a person's habits or lifestyle? These questions typify the dilemmas that are encountered at the intersection of aging and biotechnology.

The number of centenarians is increasing at a rate of about 8 percent per year in industrialized countries (Vaupel et al., 1998). Thomas Perls (chap. 8) attributes the bulk of the recent increase in lifespan to improvements in public health, such as sanitation, antibiotics, and control of conditions like high blood pressure, but he acknowledges the significance of genetics, environment, behavior, and luck. Women comprise 85 percent of centenarians, a fact that sparks some interesting speculation about biological correlates of healthy aging. Genes known to be associated with extreme old age, such as variants of apolipoprotein E and cholesteryl ester transfer protein, are the subject of intensive research and may provide clues for future antiaging interventions. Genetic links to longevity were supported by Perls's (2002) studies of 444 families, in which siblings of centenarians were found to have markedly higher relative survival probabilities at older ages and a cumulative lifelong advantage over others in their birth cohort. Perls describes a "threshold" model that can be used to explain predispositions for exceptional longevity; in this model, centenarians exceed the liability threshold for traits that lead to life-limiting illness. As Perls points out, research supports the perspective that "the older you get, the healthier you've been."

In chapter 9 Leonard Poon explores the differences between today's centenarians and the shorter-lived members of their birth cohort. Compared with younger cohorts, centenarians rarely smoked or consumed ex-cessive alcohol, and few were obese. They remained physically active and ate breakfast on a regular basis. Their diets consisted of more vitamin A and carotenoids, but they did not avoid whole milk or cholesterol-contain-ing foods. Their cognitive performance was not better than that of younger cohorts, except in the area of everyday problem solving, but educational level had a strong positive effect on level of performance. Centenarians were more dominant, suspicious, practical, and relaxed than persons in their sixties and eighties and did not report a large number of visitors to their homes except when they were sick or disabled. Centenarians did re-port somatic symptoms and some measured level of nonclinical depres-sion. Poon also looked at predictors of longevity after age 100 and found these to be social support, nourishment, cognitive skills, gender, and fam-ily longevity. Although Poon concedes that he does not have an answer to persistent questions about the key to extreme longevity, he is convinced that the human spirit and human choices supplement biological and ge-netic factors.

In chapter 10 Diane Scott-Jones critiques Perls's and Poon's findings from the perspective of developmental psychology. Both Perls and Poon acknowledged the importance of the interaction of genetic and environ-mental factors for longevity, and Scott-Jones supplements the discussion by expanding on the interactions of race, developmental variability, and societal factors in successful aging. She discusses the multiple develop-mental paths that can lead to centenarian status and proposes that sources of variability in Poon's findings include gender, region of the country, co-hort effects, selection bias, and cross-sectional study design. Scott-Jones concludes with emphasis on the impact of the dramatic social and tech-nological change that has occurred during the centenarians' lifetime and the importance of including these variables in future studies.

If centenarians exemplify successful aging, then persons with Alzheimer disease (AD) represent one example of the other extreme: aging in the con-text of dementia and loss of functional abilities. AD serves as a prototype for the progressive, unpredictable, degenerative disorders of aging. It is also a disease for which predictive genetic testing is on the horizon, a real-ity that involves the realms of genetic technology, bioethics, and clinical practice. Philibert's question about what we can do with aging becomes, What do we do with probabilistic risk information for an age-related, de-bilitating disease with no cure?

AD currently affects more than 4.5 million people in the United States, and the prevalence is predicted to triple by the year 2050 (Hebert et al., 2003). This chronic, progressive neurological disorder is characterized at first by memory impairment and reduced ability to learn, but it ultimately results in deterioration to a state of complete helplessness. Specific genes have been identified that predispose individuals to developing AD. One of these, APOE e4, confers a 3- to 15-fold increase in lifetime risk, and a blood test for this gene is available to at-risk individuals in a research setting. In chapter 11 Catherine Read and coauthors discuss the REVEAL (Risk Evaluation and Education for Alzheimer's Disease) Study, an on-going multisite randomized clinical trial designed to evaluate the psycho-logical and behavioral impact of genetic risk assessment that includes disclosure of APOE e4 status. Thus far the results of the REVEAL Study indicate that genotype information for AD can be disclosed safely and meaningfully if appropriate pre-test education and genetic counseling are provided. Nevertheless, the idea of presymptomatic genetic testing for in-curable illnesses remains controversial.

A genetic test for APOE e4 provides only probabilistic information about AD susceptibility. Potential dangers of probabilistic genetic testing for adult-onset diseases include the risk of psychological distress, family discord, insurance or employment discrimination, and social stigmatiza-tion (Green, 2002). In addition, genetic tests may confer information about first-degree relatives of the person seeking the test, and family members may not want to know this kind of risk information. Compared with the results of deterministic genetic tests (such as the one for Huntington dis-ease), which, if present, confer a 100 percent chance of ultimately devel-oping the disease, probabilistic genetic test results may be very difficult to interpret. This is further complicated by the role of environmental factors in the development of adult-onset diseases.

In chapter 12 Margaret Gatz and Jessica Brommelhoff discuss the pro-posed role of various environmental factors in the etiology of AD and the controversy about promoting unproven preventive therapies to high-risk individuals. Nongenetic factors that have been correlated with increased risk for Alzheimer disease include head trauma, microbes, toxins, and low educational level. Factors that predispose individuals to cardiovascular and cerebrovascular disease are also implicated, and this has led to promo-tion of the "heart healthy" lifestyle as a possible way to prevent or delay the onset of AD. Of greater controversy are unproven claims that medications that lower blood lipid levels, antioxidant vitamins, and cognitive exercise programs can provide protection against Alzheimer disease. As Gatz and Brommelhoff point out, "Encouraging uncorroborated prevention techniques may not only offer false hope but may also cause individuals who do develop dementia to be blamed for their condition."

In an effort to gain insight into motivation to seek presymptomatic genetic testing for AD, Ann Hurley and coauthors undertook a qualitative study of participants of the REVEAL Study. The authors discuss the results of that study and provide transcripts of some of their interviews in chapter 13. The overall findings indicate that reasons for seeking presymptomatic genetic testing for AD fall into the broad categories of learning and altruism. Learning includes the three concepts of planning, promotion, and need to know. Participation in the REVEAL Study was seen as altruistic in that it might contribute to scientific knowledge about AD. This study highlights the primacy of psychological factors in decision making about seeking genetic testing.

In chapter 14 J. Scott Roberts points out that as the clinical care of older adults increasingly includes genetic testing, practitioners must be educated about its use and limitations. In addition to knowledge about the characteristics of the specific disease and the applicable genetic tests, clinicians must consider the potential consequences of disclosing genetic information. Roberts summarizes the current literature about the impact of genetic testing for Huntington disease, cancer, and AD. For any disease, individual differences exist in information-seeking style under stress and the subsequent effects on health behavior. There are also notable differences among individuals in the ability to understand complex probabilistic information. Roberts suggests that future research about the psychological and behavioral responses to genetic testing use more appropriate outcome measures, increase sample diversity, and recognize that individual genes may affect more than one organ system.

Although we already understand a great deal about the genetic diseases associated with aging, we are only beginning to understand the impact of risk information for unpredictable scenarios and the appropriate use of genetic tests for diseases with a variable course. As Toni Miles suggests in her conclusion to part IV, primary care providers are correct to ask how knowing about a patient's genetic susceptibility will alter the medical management of a disease. In most cases it will not, but the potential effect on the family may be significant. Miles does see more immediate applicability of pharmacogenetic tests, which can help find the most effective medication for an individual based on genotype.

The chapters in part V address the larger societal contexts that influence the ethical, scientific, and practical issues at the intersection of genetics and aging. Our implicit assumptions regarding personhood, social justice, and end-of-life issues shape scientific and clinical practice and individual responses to the problems and prospects of aging in a genetically new world. Pamela Grace (chap. 16) analyzes the ethical and philosophical implications of integrating innovative biotechnology into the clinical care of older adults. She emphasizes the obligation of practitioners to have a full understanding of the technology and, more important, to consider its possible benefits and harm to an aging person with a limited ability to give informed consent. In chapter 17 Lisa Sowle Cahill and Sarah Moses present the argument that social justice demands a serious look at factors that marginalize elderly people, and they posit that genetic technologies will never be able to replace other forms of support that enhance the experience of old age and promote solidarity for the common good. Laurie Zoloth (chap. 18) uses the example of the sanitation of drinking water in the nineteenth century to illustrate the concept of resistance to new technology and compares this example with current fears about stem cell research and other genetic technologies. She examines the philosophical and theological principles that underlie the opposition to these technologies for fear of creating a society of immortal humans. Finally, in chapter 19 Rosemarie Tong reflects on the dilemmas of whole-organism human cloning, selective procreation technology, and therapies used for the purposes of enhancing oneself or one's children. She concludes that health care professionals should determine whether new technologies fall within the scope of the moral practice of medicine, and the citizenry should take responsibility for setting limits on biotechnology applications instead of waiting for controls from regulatory authorities.

Biotechnology will undoubtedly influence the future of the human species and how we age, but, as this book reveals, it is only part of a complex story. Throughout history the development of technology that is based on scientific discovery has had far-reaching effects on human society. Like the agricultural, industrial, and digital revolutions of past centuries, the current biotechnology revolution has enough general-purpose applications to have an enormous effect on individual lives, family processes, and societal practices. The biotechnology revolution may prove to be more significant than any past revolution because it has the potential to alter the essence of what it means to be human: growth, reproduction, health, and aging. Consequently, the changes we can expect from biotechnology in the future will be significantly influenced by environmental factors. Ironically, it was the reductionistic, technology-driven quest to map the human genome that led to the rejection of the concept of genetic determinism and a new appreciation for the role of the environment. Now that we know that humans have far fewer genes than the number of proteins produced, we are challenged to understand the internal and external environmental influences that mitigate when and in what form a particular protein will be made from a single gene. But the impact of the environment extends far beyond the regulation of gene expression; human growth, reproduction, health, and aging are also a function of forces of nature, local economies, regulations and policies, interpersonal relationships, societal expectations and attitudes, and resource allocation. Biotechnology in and of itself cannot revolutionize our future, and we are challenged to manage it in such a way that we ensure not only healthy aging but also self-determinism, privacy, and autonomy.

Taken together, this collection gives a complex and nuanced set of answers to Philibert's (1979) questions: Of aging, what can we know? About aging, what must we hope? With aging, what can we do? At the beginning of the twenty-first century, at the intersection of a demographic revolution and a molecular biology revolution, each of these questions requires us to reach across disciplinary and professional lines to draw on the best from philosophy, theology, medicine, life sciences, nursing, and psychology. Convening the conversation and convoying its results are a good start.

REFERENCES

Green, R. C. 2002. Risk assessment for Alzheimer's disease with genetic susceptibility testing: Has the moment arrived? *Alzheimer's Care Quarterly* 3:208–14.

Hebert, L. E., P. A. Scherr, J. L. Bienias, D. A Bennett, and D. A. Evans. 2003. Alzheimer disease in the US population: Prevalence estimates using the 2000 census. *Archives of Neurology* 60:1119–22.

Lanza, R. P., J. B Cibelli, C. Blackwell, V. J. Cristofalo, M. K. Francis, G. M. Baerlocher, et al. 2000. Extension of cell life-span and telomere length in animals
cloned from senescent somatic cells. *Science* 288:665–69.

National Center for Health Statistics. 2005. Life expectancy hits record high: Gender gap narrows. Press release, February 28.

Perls, T. T., J. Wilmoth, R. Levenson, M. Drinkwater, M. Cohen, H. Bogan, et al.
2002. Life-long sustained mortality advantage of siblings of centenarians. *Pro-
ceedings of the National Academy of Sciences of the United States of America*
99:8442–47.

Philibert, M. 1979. Philosophical approach to gerontology. In *Dimensions of Aging:
Readings,* ed. J. Hendricks and C. D. Hendricks. Pp. 379–94. Cambridge, MA:
Winthrop.

U.S. General Accounting Office. 2001. Health products for seniors: Anti-aging
products pose potential for physical and economic harm. GAO 01-1129.

Vaupel, J. W., J. R. Carey, K. Christensen, T. E. Johnson, A. I. Yashin, A. N. V. Holm,
et al. 1998. Biodemographic trajectories of longevity. *Science* 280:855–60.

CONTRIBUTORS

George J. Annas, J.D., M.P.H., Edward R. Utley Professor and Chair, Department of Health Law, Bioethics and Human Rights, Boston University School of Public Health, Boston, Massachusetts

Jessica Brommelhoff, M.A., M.P.H., Doctoral Student, Department of Psychology, University of Southern California, Los Angeles

Lisa Sowle Cahill, Ph.D., J. Donald Monan Professor of Theology, Boston College, Chestnut Hill, Massachusetts

Margaret Gatz, Ph.D., Professor, Department of Psychology, University of Southern California, Los Angeles

Pamela J. Grace, Ph D., APRN, Associate Professor of Adult Health and Ethics, Boston College Connell School of Nursing, Chestnut Hill, Massachusetts

Robert C. Green, M.D., M.P.H., Professor of Neurology, Genetics, and Epidemiology and Co-Director, Alzheimer's Disease Clinical and Research Program, Boston University Schools of Medicine and Public Health, Boston, Massachusetts

Fernando A. Guerra, M.D., M.P.H., Director of Health, San Antonio Metropolitan Health District, San Antonio, Texas

Rose M. Harvey, R.N., D.N.Sc., Adjunct Associate Professor, School of Nursing, Bouvé College of Health Sciences, Northeastern University, Boston, Massachusetts

Kathy J. Horvath, Ph.D., R.N., Associate Director for Education and Evaluation, New England Geriatric Research Education and Clinical Center, E. N. Rogers Memorial Veterans Hospital, Bedford, Massachusetts

Ann C. Hurley, R.N., D.N.Sc., FAAN, Senior Nurse Scientist Emerita, Center for Nursing Excellence, Brigham and Women's Hospital, Boston, Massachusetts

Robert Lanza, M.D., Vice President of Research and Scientific Development, Advanced Cell Technology, Worcester, Massachusetts; Adjunct Professor, Institute of Regenerative Medicine, Wake Forest University School of Medicine, Winston-Salem, North Carolina

Karen Lebacqz, Ph.D., Robert Gordon Sproul Professor of Theological Ethics Emerita, Pacific School of Religion, Berkeley, California; former Bioethicist in Residence, Yale University, New Haven, Connecticut

Erin Linnenbringer, M.S., CGC, Doctoral Student, Department of Health Behavior and Health Education, University of Michigan School of Public Health, Ann Arbor

Maxwell J. Mehlman, J.D., Arthur E. Petersilge Professor of Law, Case Western Reserve University School of Law, and Professor of Biomedical Ethics, Case Western Reserve University School of Medicine, Cleveland, Ohio

Toni P. Miles, M.D., Ph.D., Wise-Nelson Chair and Clinical Geriatrics Research Professor, Department of Family and Geriatric Medicine, University of Louisville, Louisville, Kentucky

Sarah Moses, Ph.D.(c), Teaching Fellow, Department of Theology, Boston College, Chestnut Hill, Massachusetts

Thomas T. Perls, M.D., M.P.H., Director, New England Centenarian Study, Associate Professor of Medicine and Geriatrics, Boston University Medical Center, Boston, Massachusetts

Leonard W. Poon, Ph.D., Professor of Psychology, Chair, Faculty of Gerontology, and Director, Gerontology Center, University of Georgia, Athens

Catherine Y. Read, Ph.D., R.N., Associate Professor of Adult Health, Boston College Connell School of Nursing, Chestnut Hill, Massachusetts

J. Scott Roberts, Ph.D., Assistant Professor, Department of Health Behavior and Health Education, University of Michigan School of Public Health, Ann Arbor

Diane Scott-Jones, Ph.D., Professor, Department of Psychology, Boston College, Chestnut Hill, Massachusetts

Thomas A. Shannon, Ph.D., Professor Emeritus of Religion and Social Ethics, Department of Humanities and Arts, Worcester Polytechnic Institute, Worcester, Massachusetts

Richard L. Sprott, Ph.D., Executive Director, The Ellison Medical Foundation, Bethesda, Maryland

Rosemarie Tong, Ph.D., Distinguished Professor in Health Care Ethics and Director, Center for Professional and Applied Ethics, Department of Philosophy, University of North Carolina at Charlotte

Laurie Zoloth, Ph.D., Professor of Medical Humanities and Bioethics and of Religion and Director, Center for Bioethics, Science, and Society, Northwestern University Feinberg School of Medicine, Chicago, Illinois

PART 1

INTRODUCTION

Reality Check

What Is Genetic Research on Aging Likely to Produce, and What Are the Ethical and Clinical Implications of Those Advances?

RICHARD L. SPROTT, PH.D.

Longevity and Its Effects on the Burden of Disease

By 2030 the number of people in the United States aged 65 or older is likely to double. This increase is due to both population increase and increased longevity. Life expectancy at birth in the United States in 1900 was 49.2 years. By 2000 this figure had grown to 76.9 years, and now it is 77.6 years (white females, 80.5; white males, 75.4; black females, 76.1; black males, 69.2; NCHS, 2005). Currently, life expectancy at birth in the United States is increasing by roughly two-tenths of a year each year. As a result, life expectancy by 2030 could easily reach 82 or more years (more for women and a bit less for men), not 100 or 150 years, as some in the media would have us believe.

An obvious concern is how this increase in the number of older Americans will play out in terms of opportunity and burden. What will the balance be? Can anything we do now have a significant effect on what happens over the next two or three decades? The answers to these questions are of enormous consequence to us all, and what most Americans believe is based on a much-distorted presentation of the issues by elements of our culture with divergent agendas.

Political Interests have a stake in presenting the data in ways that can be used to generate support for action. Thus, we hear that because of longer lives, Social Security "needs to be reformed," or will be broke by 2010, or is safe until 2050, or can be saved if we make one or another change. My aim here is not to argue which of these views is right or wrong, but to point out that it is little wonder that the average American is bewildered. It makes sense to obtain the best possible data to inform policy makers so that decision making can be based on fact, not political expediency, even though we all recognize that facts are inconvenient in political discussion.

On the other hand, the antiaging/nutriceutical industry has a stake in presenting a dreadful image of "normal aging" in conjunction with touting the wonders of current and developing therapies. This set of interests is divided into two major camps. One camp, the real scientists (including many of my scientific colleagues), predicts that research will produce significant increases in longevity with concomitant increases in "health span," if we will just provide the needed funds. The other camp, the hucksters, proclaims that great increases in individual longevity are already possible if individuals will just buy the appropriate drugs, nutritional supplements, hormone therapies, spa treatments, or all of these together. The cost of the hucksters' claims is twofold: they encourage the belief that health is something that comes out of a bottle rather than a result of genes interacting with healthy lifestyles, and the therapies themselves often cost enormous amounts of cold hard cash. Even if they worked, they would be available only to the very rich.

Real research, with animal model systems in which increases in longevity have actually been achieved, so far shows that increased longevity does not increase disability. The age-dependent diseases to which these animals (rodents, flies, worms, and maybe monkeys) are susceptible occur later in life, and the period of compromised health is about the same. Two decades ago there was a spirited debate about whether increased lifespan in humans would or would not lead to great increases in disability. So far we have not seen an increase of this kind. We do see more cancer and dementia now than in the early decades of the last century, as many more people live long enough to succumb to late-life disease. There is no reason to expect, however, that there are diseases we know nothing about waiting to manifest in centenarians.

In the long run, the question is not whether greater longevity will result in a greater health burden but rather what sorts of improvement can we realistically expect research to provide to an aging population that will reduce the burden of disease. These changes could easily compensate for the expected increases in the numbers of aged individuals.

The Success of Research on the Horizon

We are in the midst of the most exciting and important scientific era in the history of the world. I finished graduate school 40 years ago, and virtually everything I do scientifically today is the result of discoveries made since then. Many of the important discoveries for aging are the product of research undertaken in the last decade. The pace of discovery is increasing at dizzying speed. While this is sometimes disconcerting, the opportunities for improving the human condition are mind boggling even without having to imagine 150- or 500-year-old humans.

The completion of the human genome project has given us the tools to understand how our genes interact with our environment (including lifestyle) to affect how long and how well we live. While I don't think we are going to see 150-year-old humans anytime soon, I do believe that we will find new, effective therapies for age-related diseases. Drugs will be designed to match our genetic makeup so that they are both more effective and less likely to have adverse side effects. For some diseases we will be able to provide replacement genes or gene products to compensate for our own "defective" genes.

The basic research that underlies these possibilities is providing understanding of the myriad ways our bodily systems interact. For example, research on how telomeres might determine the lifespan of cells connects with research on the involvement of telomeres in cancer and may explain the strong link between aging and cancer.

Let me expand briefly on the telomere example, as it nicely illustrates the potential of modern genetic research. Telomeres are DNA sequences at the ends of chromosomes. This description is an oversimplification of the relationship of telomeres to aging, but it does suggest how telomeres, aging, and cancer might be interrelated. In 1965 Leonard Hayflick discovered that cells growing in culture had a limited lifespan. After approximately 50 population doublings, the cells in the culture stopped dividing and entered a "senescent" state. There was at the time great hope that if we could understand this cell senescence, we would unlock the secrets of aging. The key questions were how a cell culture can count its divisions, and why reaching some number of divisions (like 50) will result in senescence.

Years passed with no apparent progress toward answering those questions. Then Blackburn and Gall (1978) showed that when cells divide, telomeres shorten because of what is known as the "end replication" problem. This shortening is often compared to removing beads from a string of beads as pieces of DNA drop off at each division. Whether telomere shortening actually leads to senescence has been the subject of nearly endless controversy. Adding DNA at the end of telomeres appeared to stabilize cells and prevent cell senescence. While this might explain how a cell culture could "count," it did not explain why telomere shortening would result in senescence. Then in 1999 Titia de Lange and Jack Griffith (Griffith et al., 1999) showed that telomeres are not linear ends of the chromosome but are actually loops, which they called t-loops. At each division, when DNA is removed, the loop becomes a little smaller and tighter. Eventually it is possible that there is not enough DNA left to form a loop, the loop breaks, and the cell repair mechanisms read this as DNA damage and push the cell into senescence. Providing telomerase to the cells prevents telomere shortening and senescence.

Many tumors are composed of immortal cells. In fact, immortality at the cell level results in death of the host organism. These cells appear to become immortal when DNA damage results in the loss of senescence capability. While normal differentiated cells do not have active telomerase, most tumor cells do. The possibilities that arise from these observations are staggering. Manipulation of telomerase levels could conceivably be used to produce long life by adding telomerase to some cells or to provide a silver bullet for cancer by removing telomerase from tumor cells.

One outcome of increases in our knowledge will be a better "health span." Another will surely be increases in hype, charlatanism, media confusion, and policy controversy. We can view our aging population as a collection of "greedy geezers," as a source of wisdom, or as something in between. It is in the best interest of all us that we begin now to discuss what is realistically possible and how we will deal with the inevitable effects on our society. What we do now will have an impact on what happens and how it affects our lives. The changes are coming. We can either meet them prepared or let them overwhelm us.

Ethical Implications

Any ethical discussion of the potential effects of genetic research on aging must start with the recognition that what we ought to do and what we are likely to do are two quite different things. No amount of discussion or moral suasion will prevent lifespan extension or immortality research. Likewise, we are not likely to stop the purveyors of elixirs, real or ersatz, from selling their wares to the desperate and gullible. With that caveat, I think some of the more important ethical issues are well known. Some of these issues were nicely enunciated in Daniel Callahan's 1987 book *Setting Limits*. Callahan's views still resonate with many of those who oppose lifespan extension or "prolongevity." His major points include the following:

1. "Medicine should be used to allow achievement of a 'natural and fitting' lifespan and the relief of suffering" (53). Many others argue that we do not know what a "natural and fitting" lifespan is. Scientific beliefs on this issue depend heavily on one's assumptions about the underlying causes of aging and death. If one believes that there are basic processes of aging, then it follows that there is something like a "natural" lifespan. If, on the other hand, one believes that aging is the consequence of the effects of disease and wear and tear, then it follows that eliminating those effects will produce a very different "natural" lifespan.

2. "There are better ways to spend money than indefinitely extending lifespan" (53). Here many will argue that Callahan poses a straw man. There are many other options than "indefinite lifespan extension." Furthermore, money spent on improving health as a means of extending lifespan will still have an effect on health.

3. "If concepts such as 'old,' 'aging,' and 'premature death' are a function of the state-of-the-art of medicine at any given moment, then it is hard to imagine a solid basis for determining what health demands, expectations, or desires on the part of the elderly are reasonable or unreasonable" (56). This is not a problem of aging. It is hard to imagine what health demands on the part of *anyone* in our society are reasonable or unreasonable. Why should elderly people be any different? To take a position that they are is to join those who feel that we should not "waste" resources on those who have already lived a

full life, the "greedy geezers." This view makes great sense when we look at individuals who seem to be just "taking up space" and no sense at all when we look at vibrant late-life achievers.

A nice example of the latter is provided by Callahan in his discussion of the views of Matilda and John Riley (73). In their 1986 *Daedalus* article they say, "It is clear that increased longevity: (1) prolongs the opportunity for accumulating social, psychological, and biological experiences; (2) maximizes a person's opportunities to complete or to change the role assignments of early and middle life—for example, to change jobs, marriage partners, or educational plans, and to take on new roles in the later years; (3) prolongs a person's relationships to others—to spouse, parents, offspring, friends—whose lives are extended; and (4) increases the potential structural complexity of a person's social networks—for example, of kinship, friendship, community—as all members survive longer."

That is a fine example of the way John and Matilda lived life. The Rileys were invariably optimistic and lived to ripe old ages. John died in 2002 and Matilda in 2004, both at the age of 93. Matilda was a fine exemplar of productive old age, but I think she was also a prime example of the "blame the victim" school of thought about disability in old age. By that I do not mean that she necessarily thought that disabled elderly people were always personally responsible for their disability, but rather that many could surely do better if they would but try. That view is probably shared by many people, and therein lies an ethical dilemma. It is true that we seem to "waste" resources on people who choose to "vegetate." But how are we to decide who is worthy and who is not? By whom, and on the basis of what criteria, should such decisions be made? Should we deny resources to those who don't take care of themselves? Or should we deny resources to very old, disabled people?

This question of resource allocation is *the* central ethical question we face in this discussion. At bottom, the issue is not age. Age is just one of the markers we use to discriminate when we allocate resources of any type, including the benefits of scientific advances and expensive medical treatments. Ultimately, the question is how we will allocate the great opportunities we will see as a result of a better understanding of our biology, not whether we can stop that progress.

REFERENCES

Blackburn, E. H., and J. C. Gall. 1978. A tandemly repeated sequence at the termini of the extrachromosomal ribosomal RNA genes in Tetrahymena. *Journal of Molecular Biology* 120:33–53.

Callahan, D. 1987. *Setting Limits: Medical Goals in an Aging Society.* New York: Simon and Schuster.

Griffith, J. D., L. Comeau, S. Rosenfield, R. M. Stansel, A.Bianchi, H. Moss, and T. de Lange. 1999. Mammalian telomeres end in a large duplex loop. *Cell* 97: 503–14.

Hayflick, L. 1965. The limited in vitro lifetime of human diploid cell strains. *Experimental Cell Research* 57:614–36.

National Center for Health Statistics. 2005. Life expectancy hits record high: Gender gap narrows. Press release, February 28.

Riley, M. W., and J. W. Riley Jr. 1986. Longevity and social structure: The added years. *Daedalus* 115:53–54.

CHAPTER 2

Meeting the Challenges
of a Diverse Aging Society

FERNANDO A. GUERRA, M.D., M.P.H.

Addressing the issue of aging in contemporary society is a complex and challenging exercise—an exercise that is obviously demanding more and more of our time and attention. This is due in part to the fact that persons 65 years of age or older are recognized as the fastest-growing segment of our population. The Centers for Disease Control and Prevention (2007) point out that by 2030, this group of older Americans will have doubled to 71 million, or one in every five Americans. We also must recognize that this is an increasingly diverse group. They range from the relatively healthy and active "young oldsters," to frail and impaired persons in their eighties, to a growing number of centenarians. There are also important racial, ethnic, and gender variations to consider, as well as significant cultural issues to address as more and more immigrants find their way to our shores and borders. Persons aging within different cultures have different needs, experience aging in different ways, and even have vastly different perceptions of what constitutes good health and acceptable health care. These projections mean that our existing service delivery systems for public health, medical care, and social welfare services, already strained, will be placed under even greater stress. These abstract demographics will play themselves out in real-life scenarios that will affect the quality of life of individual older Americans as well as our capacity as a nation to face up to the difficult choices that lie ahead. This may well be a defining moment in the evolution of our national character and identity. The task is to focus our creativity, commitment, and sense of traditional social values to a search for a balanced, sensitive, and humane resolution to these challenges.

Aging is not just a process that can be measured or a population that can be counted, plotted, and tracked. It is also a reality that will be experienced by most of us. A growing segment of our nation is living out this experience for longer and longer periods of time. This is largely uncharted territory. We have not really had to face these new realities before. In earlier times people didn't live long enough to suffer the burden of chronic disease or experience the debilitating effects of arthritis, Alzheimer disease, and other degenerative conditions. The family was the primary caregiver, and the multigenerational unit provided for the material, social, psychological, and spiritual need of its members. That role has been largely abdicated. The twenty-first century is ushering in an era in which roles, responsibilities, relationships, and societal expectations are rapidly being transformed. This paradigm shift is being felt throughout society but is especially visible and dramatic in its manifestations when we consider its impact on the elderly. When we view elderly people through the prism of health, even more variables are introduced. What are the special needs of this population? What kinds of services should we develop that will best address these needs? Are the traditional venues for service delivery such as physicians' offices, clinics, and hospitals the best or only options? Who will be delivering this care? What kind of health care workforce do we need to train? Beyond demographics and health statistics, however, we must also engage the broader challenges of poverty, access to care, and the maintenance and defense of our existing safety net through political action and advocacy. We have already increasingly seen the evolution of a two-tier system of health care. The prospect of a growing population of elderly, many of whom will have limited means, requiring expensive new treatments and interventions while at the same time threatened with cutbacks in existing entitlement programs, runs the risk of taking us further down that road.

Ethical considerations around resource allocation, appropriate treatment options, and control of decision making further complicate the final years and the final days of life for both the family and caregivers of the elderly.

In some ways we can be seen as victims of our own success. Increased longevity is largely due to the contributions and accomplishments of public health over the years. The cumulative impact of our success in providing pure water, clean air, safe food, health screenings, immunizations, and control of communicable diseases cannot be overstated. Aggressive public education campaigns have also had a positive impact. Promotion of smoking cessation, nutrition, exercise, and weight control is increasingly finding receptive audiences. Combined with the significant advances in research, pharmaceuticals, and medical technologies, such accomplishments mean that many more of us will experience longer life expectancies.

Will those years be healthier, happier, and more productive as a result of our advances, or will we fall victim to the "law of unintended consequences"? Quality of life may suffer, health disparities may increase, and intergenerational competition may surface. There are no clear solutions to many of these dilemmas at this time. Some of our finest minds, however, are engaged in thoughtful consideration of these issues, and new insights and analysis are resulting in a growing public awareness of the scope and scale of the challenge that confronts us. A comparison of the disease profiles for 1900 and 2000 is informative. In the beginning of the twentieth century, pneumonia, influenza, tuberculosis, and diarrhea were the major causes of death. As we enter the twenty-first century, these causes of death have been replaced by heart disease, cancer, and cerebrovascular complications. Our growing aging population will be especially vulnerable and at risk under this scenario. We are confident, however, that public health can make similar contributions in this new environment. Our traditional strengths in prevention, education, and early intervention will be central to this effort. Public health has a long history and a strong record in this regard.

One of our traditional public health functions and responsibilities has been to assess the community's health status and monitor those indicators that reflect it. Accurate descriptions of the needs and characteristics of our older adults will be essential to plan appropriate strategies and identify necessary resources. We have grown increasingly sophisticated in this regard in recent years, and our new analytical tools have allowed us to examine the relationships and interplay of socioeconomic, psychological, and environmental forces in more detail. This kind of assessment provides us with the data and insights that in turn can inform and shape the societal dialogue that must take place as we prepare to engage these issues.

Another core public health function involves developing policy recommendations based on those assessments. Just as public health helped create new agendas for the fields of women's health, children's health, and minority health, so will it embrace the challenge of developing a new conceptual model that will define the characteristics, health needs, and treatment strategies most relevant to this special population. Meaningful change can occur when our energies are focused, our priorities clear, and our commitment strong. We need to muster the kind of groundswell of support that greeted the promulgation of the Children's Charter in the 1930s. President Herbert Hoover assembled leaders in the medical, educational, and social development fields as they touch on the life of children to study the needs of children and to make recommendations for their care and protection. Fifteen basic recommendations emerged from these deliberations, and they provided the foundation and framework for a series of progressive and humane measures that grew over the intervening decades to shape the safety net that protects our children to this day. Only an endeavor of similar scale and scope will allow us to focus public policy, priorities, and resources on support of our older adults.

While we are continually improving the design of our system and the quality of its products, the "gap widens," as not all of our citizens benefit equally from that progress. Health disparities are defined as the unequal distribution of health care services among groups or the disproportionate representation of illness or disease among such groups. These include not only racial and ethnic categories but also those defined by socioeconomic status, age, gender, or even geographical location. In an environment in which Medicare and Medicaid are targeted for cutbacks, those least able to protect current entitlements are children, disabled people, and the elderly. The more affluent, educated, and politically active are better positioned to protect their interests. An important responsibility of those in the field of public health is to provide assurances that every person, regardless of income or condition, has access to at least the most basic level of health care.

The anticipated size of our aging population in the next few decades and the nature of the chronic diseases that will need to be managed will test and strain any system that we might design. It will be increasingly important that public health have a seat at the table as we attempt to address and resolve these difficult and complex new challenges. The public health system's perspective and competencies allow us to track trends, document disparities, identify unmet needs, and advocate for the kind of safety net needed to protect this sometimes "invisible" population. Public health has had a long and successful track record of informing, involving, and motivating critical community stakeholders with respect to difficult and contentious issues such as resource allocation, including facilities and the personnel to meet the needs of those most vulnerable.

Public health also brings a special sensitivity to the social determinants of health, an especially critical dimension for this constituency. It is alert to the subtle demographic shifts that are changing the population profiles of many of our large urban centers across the nation. Many of these communities are experiencing significant growth in their immigrant populations and the higher birth rates that often accompany this phenomenon. Communities facing this kind of growth, coupled with the longer life expectancies of their older residents, will face difficult decisions as they attempt to balance conflicting needs in an environment of limited or diminishing resources. These issues grow even more complex when we factor in the aging members of our undocumented population who are routinely denied access to the most basic of our geriatric services and programs.

We must vigorously resist any attempt to weaken or reduce the hard-won protections that are currently in place. Public health will need to forge new and more effective linkages with the private sector as well as other community interest groups to create strong, active, and vocal constituencies that can influence legislative agendas and allocation of resources for pursuing these goals. Although we are confident in the final triumph of hope over adversity, this will not come easily. We must remind ourselves that ultimately, any success we realize will accrue not only to our own benefit but also to the benefit of our children and grandchildren in generations to come.

REFERENCE

Centers for Disease Control and Prevention. 2007. *The State of Aging and Health in America 2007*. Whitehouse Station, NJ: Merck Company Foundation. www .cdc.gov/aging.

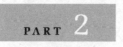
PART 2

IMMORTALITY

CHAPTER 3

Immortality through Cloning?

Reproduction, Regeneration, and the Posthuman

GEORGE J. ANNAS, J.D., M.P.H.

We humans tend to worry first about ourselves, next about our families, then about our communities.[1] In times of great stress, such as war or natural disaster, we may focus temporarily on our country. But we almost never think about our planet as a whole or the human species as a whole. This constricted perspective, perhaps best exemplified by the American consumer, has led to the environmental degradation of the earth, a gross and widening gap in living standards between rich and poor nations and peoples, and a scientific research agenda that focuses almost exclusively on the needs and desires of the wealthy West. Reversing worldwide trends toward market-based atomization and increasing indifference to the suffering of others will require a human rights focus forged by the development of what Vaclav Havel termed a "species consciousness."

In this chapter I explore human cloning and inheritable genetic alterations from the perspective of the human species and human rights and contrast that perspective with the much more narrow view of individuals who seek to use these technologies to radically alter their characteristics, including the length of life. In this context I also suggest language for a proposed international "Convention on the Preservation of the Human Species" that would outlaw all efforts to initiate a pregnancy using either intentionally modified genetic material or human replication cloning, such as through somatic cell nuclear transfer. I summarize recent international legal action in these areas, relate these actions to arguments for and against a treaty, and conclude with some suggestions for further action.

Human Rights and the Human Species

The deployment of the atomic bomb not only presented the world for the first time with the prospect of total annihilation but also, paradoxically, led to a renewed emphasis on the nuclear family, complete with its personal bomb shelter. The conclusion of World War II (with the dropping of the only two atomic bombs ever used in war) led to the recognition that world wars were now suicidal and to the formation of the United Nations with the primary goal of preventing such wars. That we are all fundamentally the same, all human, with the same dignity and rights, is at the core of the United Nations Charter and the Universal Declaration of Human Rights.

Membership in the human species is central to the meaning and enforcement of human rights, and respect for basic human rights is essential for the survival of the human species. The development of the concept of crimes against humanity was a milestone for universalizing human rights in that it recognized that there were certain actions, such as slavery and genocide, that implicated the entire species and so merited universal condemnation (Bassiouni, 1992). Nuclear weapons were immediately recognized as a technology that requires international control, and extreme genetic manipulations like cloning and inheritable genetic alteration are similar. Both belong in the general category of species-endangering activities. In fact, cloning and inheritable genetic alterations can be seen as crimes against humanity of a unique sort: techniques that can alter the essence of humanity itself (and thus threaten to change the foundation of human rights as well) by taking human evolution into our own hands and directing it toward the development of a new species, sometimes termed the posthuman.[2] It may be that species-altering techniques, like cloning and inheritable genetic modifications, could provide benefits to the human species in extraordinary circumstances. For example, asexual genetic replication could potentially save humans from extinction if all humans were rendered sterile by some catastrophic event, transforming an otherwise species-endangering activity into a species-saving one.

As a baseline, if we take human rights and democracy seriously, a decision to alter a fundamental beneficial characteristic of humans should not be taken by any individual or corporation without wide discussion among all members of the affected population. No individual scientist or corporation has the moral warrant to redesign humans (any more than any individual scientist or corporation has the moral warrant to design a new, lethal virus or bacterium that could kill large numbers of humans). Species-endangering activities directly concern all humans and should be decided on only democratically by a body that is representative of everyone on the planet. These are the most important decisions we will ever make. The widespread condemnation of human replicative cloning by governments around the world provides a perhaps unique opportunity for the world to begin to work together to take some control over the biotechnology that threatens our very existence.

The environmental movement has adopted the precautionary principle to help stem the tide of environmental alterations that are detrimental to humans. One version of this principle holds that "when an activity raises threats of harm to human health or the environment . . . the proponent of that activity, rather than the public, should bear the burden of proof [that the activity is more likely to be beneficial than harmful]."[3] The only way to shift the burden of proof is to outlaw dangerous and potentially lethal activities, thus requiring their proponents to change the law before proceeding. This can be done nation by nation but can be effective only by means of an internationally enforceable ban (because scientists and laboratories can move from country to country). The actual text of a treaty banning human replicative cloning and inheritable modifications is and will continue to be the subject of international debate. Following a national conference, "Beyond Cloning," held at Boston University in 2001, Lori Andrews and I suggested the following language (obviously subject to negotiation and added details) as a basis for going forward.[4]

Convention on the Preservation of the Human Species

The Parties to this Convention,

Noting that the Charter of the United Nations affirms human rights, based on the dignity and worth of the human person and on equal rights of all persons,

Noting that the Universal Declaration of Human Rights affirms the principle of the inadmissibility of discrimination,

Realizing that human dignity and human rights derive from our common humanity,

Noting the increased power of genetic science, which opens up vast prospects for improving health, but also has the power to fundamentally diminish humanity by producing a child through human cloning or through intentionally producing an inheritable genetic change,

Concerned that human cloning, which for the first time would produce children with predetermined genotypes, rather than novel genotypes, might cause these children to be deprived of their human rights,

Concerned that by altering fundamental human characteristics even to the extent of possibly producing a new human species or subspecies, genetic science will cause the resulting persons to be treated unequally or deprived of their human rights,

Recognizing the history of abuses of human rights in the name of genetic science,

Believing that no individual, nation, or corporation has the moral or legal warrant to engage in species-altering procedures, including cloning and genetic alteration of reproductive cells or embryos for the creation of a child,

Believing that the creation of a new species or subspecies of humans could easily lead to genocide or slavery,

Stressing the need for global cooperation to prevent the misuse of genetic science in ways that undermine human dignity and human rights,

Have agreed on the following:

Article 1

Parties shall take all reasonable action, including the adoption of criminal laws, to prohibit anyone from initiating or attempting to initiate a human pregnancy or other form of gestation using embryos or reproductive cells which have undergone intentional inheritable genetic modification.

Article 2

Parties shall take all reasonable action, including the adoption of criminal laws, to prohibit anyone from using somatic cell nuclear transfer or any other cloning technique for the purpose of initiating or attempting to initiate a human pregnancy or other form of gestation.

Article 3

Parties shall implement a system of national oversight through legislation, executive order, decree, or other mechanism to regulate facilities engaged in assisted human reproduction or otherwise using human gametes or embryos for experimentation or clinical purposes to ensure that such facilities meet informed consent, safety, and ethical standards.

Article 4

A Conference of the Parties and a Secretariat shall be established to oversee implementation of the Convention.

Article 5

Reservations to this Convention are not permitted.

Article 6

For the purpose of this Convention, the term "somatic cell nuclear transfer" shall mean transferring the nucleus of a human somatic cell into an ovum or oocyte. "Somatic cell" shall mean any cell of a human embryo, fetus, child or adult other than a reproductive cell. "Embryo" shall include a fertilized egg, zygote (including a blastomere and blastocyst), and preembryo. "Reproductive cell" shall mean a human gamete and its precursors.

Perhaps the most difficult challenge in implementing this treaty is setting up the monitoring and enforcement mechanisms. The Article 4 process would have to address these. In general terms, monitoring and compliance bodies must be broadly representative, possess authority to oversee activities related to cloning and human genetic modification, and be able to enforce bans by announcing and denouncing potential violators. It also seems reasonable to support the establishment of two new international crimes: initiation of a pregnancy to create a human clone and initiation of a pregnancy using a genetically altered embryo.

Why an International Convention?

On the tenth anniversary of the cloning of Dolly the sheep, *Nature* editorialized that cloning could be an acceptable way to have babies for those people for whom it is "the only means to bypass sterility or genetic disease" and that "unless there is some unknown fundamental biological obstacle, and given wholly positive ethical motivations, human reproductive cloning is an eventual certainty" (*Nature*, 2007). [5] Is humanity really so helpless and fatalistic when confronted by technologies that could change the very definition of what it means to be human? What have we learned since Dolly's birth?

First, virtually every scientist in the world with an opinion believes it is unsafe to attempt a human pregnancy with a cloned embryo. This is, for example, the unanimous conclusion of a 2002 report from the U.S. National Academy of Sciences, which recommended that human "reproductive" cloning be outlawed in the United States. [6] Although scientists seldom like to predict the future without overwhelming data to support them, many believe human cloning or inheritable genetic alternations at the embryo level will never be safe because they will always be inherently unpredictable in their effects on the children and their offspring. As embryologist Stewart Newman noted, for example, it is unlikely that a human created from the union of "two damaged cells" (an enucleated egg and a nucleus removed from a somatic cell) could ever be healthy. [7] Of course, adding genetic modification to the somatic cell's nucleus adds another series of events that could go wrong, because genes will seldom have a single function but will interact in complex and unpredictable ways with other genes. [8] It is worth underlining that the dangers are not only physical but also psychological. Whether cloned children could ever overcome the psychological problems associated with their origins is unknown and perhaps unknowable. [9] In short, the safety concerns, which make attempts to clone or genetically alter a human being inherently unethical human experiments, provide sufficient scientific justification for the treaty.

If and when safety can be assured, assuming this will ever be possible, two primary arguments have been put forth in favor of proceeding with cloning (and its first cousin, inheritable genetic alterations): cloning is a type of human reproduction that can help infertile couples have genetically related children, and cloning is a part of human "progress" (potentially leading to a new type of genetic immortality), so to prevent it is to be antiscientific.

The infertility argument is made by physiologist Panos Zavos and his former colleague, Italian infertility specialist Severino Antinori. They argue that the inability of a sterile male to have a genetically related child is such a human tragedy that it justifies human cloning. [10] This view not only ignores the rights and interests of women and children (even if only males are to be cloned, the eggs must be procured from a woman, the embryos are gestated by a woman, and the child is the subject of the experiment) but also contains a highly contested assertion: that asexual genetic replication or duplication should be seen as human reproduction.[11] In fact, humans are a sexually reproducing species and have never reproduced or replicated themselves asexually.

Asexual replication may or may not be categorized by future courts as a form of human reproduction, but there are strong arguments against it. First, asexual reproduction displaces a fundamental characteristic of what it means to be human (a sexually reproducing species) by making sexual reproduction involving the genetic mixture of male and female gametes optional. Second, the "child" in an asexual replication is also the twin brother of the male "parent," a relationship that has never existed before in human society. The first clone, for example, will be the first human being with a single genetic "parent" (unless his biological grandparents are taken to be the actual "parents" of the clone). Third, the genetic replica of a genetically sterile man is himself sterile and can "reproduce" only by cloning. This means either that infertility is not a major problem (because if it was, it would be unethical for a physician intentionally to create a child with this problem) or that the desire of existing adults should take precedent over the welfare of children. Neither conclusion is persuasive, and this is probably why, although some ethicists believe that cloning could be considered a form of human reproduction, infertility specialists have not joined Antinori's call for human cloning as a treatment for infertile males. In fact, the organization that represents infertility specialists in the United States, and which is generally opposed to regulation of infertility treatment, the American Society of Reproductive Medicine, has consistently opposed human cloning.[12]

There are, nonetheless, legal commentators who believe that human cloning should be classified as a form of human reproduction and be constitutionally protected as such, at least if it is the only way for an individual to have a "genetically related child." The strongest proponent of this view is probably John Robertson (1999), although Ronald Dworkin (2000, 437–42) shares his enthusiasm. It is unclear that human reproduction or procreation of a kind protected by principles of autonomy and self-fulfillment can be found in a "right to have a genetically related child." As Leon Kass noted in another context (1985, 110–11), it cannot be just the genetic tie that is important in human reproduction, because if it was, this could be accomplished by having one's twin brother have a child with one's wife—the genetic tie would be identical, yet few, if any, would argue that this method of reproduction should satisfy the twin's right to have a "genetically related child." Moreover, in cloning, the *genetic* relationship is not a parent-child relationship at all, but a sibling relationship. Genes are important, but there is more to human reproduction, as protected by the United States Constitution, than simple genetic replication.

The second major argument in favor of human cloning is, as the title of this chapter implies, that it can produce a form of immortality. This is the premise of the Raelian cult, which has formed its own corporation, Clonaid, to engage in human cloning. The leader of the cult, who calls himself Rael (formerly Claude Vorilhon, the editor of a French motor sport magazine), believes that all humans were created in the laboratories of the planet Elohim, and that the Elohims have instructed Rael and his followers to develop cloning on Earth to provide earthlings with a form of immortality (Rael, 1998).[13] The Raelians, of course, can believe whatever they want to believe. But just as human sacrifice has been outlawed, so too can experiments that pose a significant danger to women and children, and the religious beliefs of this cult do not provide a sufficient justification to refrain from outlawing cloning.

Two basic arguments about the future regulation of these technologies have also emerged. The first, exemplified by Lee Silver, is that these technologies, while not necessarily desirable, are unstoppable because the market combined with parental desire will drive scientists and physicians to offer these services to demanding couples. As parents now seek early educational enrichment for their children, parents of the future will seek early genetic enhancement to give them a competitive advantage in life. Silver (1997) believes this will ultimately lead to the creation of two separate species or subspecies, the GenRich and "the naturals."[14]

A related "do nothing" argument is that regulation may not be needed because the technologies will not be widely used. The thought is that humans may muddle through either because the science of human genetic alterations may never prove possible, or because it will be used by only a handful of humans because most will instinctively reject it. Steven Pinker is probably the most articulate spokesperson for this view. He argues (2003) that at least as long as genetic engineering of children remains a risky business, few parents will actually be willing to risk the health of their future children for a speculative genetic improvement. Pinker may be correct, but he may not be. In any event, his arguments do not obviate the desirability of a democratically formed regulatory scheme.[15]

The primary arguments against cloning and inheritable genetic alterations are that these interventions would require massive dangerous and unethical human experimentation;[16] that cloning would inevitably be bad for the resulting children by restricting their liberty (Jonas, 1974); that cloning would lead to a new eugenics movement for "designer children" (because if an individual could pick the entire genome of their future child, it would seem impossible to prohibit individuals from picking specific genetic characteristics);[17] and that it would likely lead to the creation of a new species or subspecies of humans, the posthuman.[18] In the context of the species, the last argument has received the least attention, and so it is worth saying more about what the creation of a posthuman would mean.

The core argument is that cloning will inevitably lead to attempts to modify the somatic cell nucleus to create not genetic duplicates of existing people but "better" children.[19] This attempt will either succeed or fail. If it fails, that is the end of it. If it succeeds, however, something like the scenario envisioned by Silver and others, such as Nancy Kress, will unfold: a new species or subspecies of humans will emerge.[20] The new species, or posthumans, will likely view the old normal humans as inferiors, even savages, fit for slavery or slaughter. The normals, on the other hand, may see the posthumans as a threat and, if they can, engage in a preemptive strike by killing the posthumans before they themselves are killed or enslaved by them.

The predictable potential for genocide, which I have termed "genetic genocide," makes species-altering experiments potential weapons of mass destruction and makes the unaccountable genetic engineer a potential bioterrorist. This is why cloning and genetic modification is of specieswide concern and why an international treaty to address this species-endangering activity is called for. Such a treaty is necessary because existing laws on cloning and germline genetic alterations, even though often well intentioned, have serious limitations.[21] Some are mere moratoria and have already expired. Some are limited as to the type of species-altering technologies they ban, covering only cloning and not germline genetic interventions, or even just applying to cloning via a limited range of techniques. Some of the existing laws have also been outpaced by technology and do not apply to comprehensively ban all forms of reproductive cloning and germline interventions. Others are ambiguous about what they cover. In some cases, potentially relevant laws were adopted more than two decades ago to deal with a different set of technologies and concerns; it is unclear whether their expansive prohibitions will be applied to the newer technologies of reproductive cloning and germline intervention. Moreover, many of the existing declarations and laws do not include appropriate sanctions. And, of course, scientists can readily cross national borders to do their research in another country without a prohibition.[22]

Numerous international entities have called for an enforceable ban on species-altering interventions. The World Health Organization at its 51st World Health Assembly reaffirmed that "cloning for replication of human beings is ethically unacceptable and contrary to human dignity and integrity." WHO urges member states to "foster continued and informed debate on these issues and to take appropriate steps, including legal and juridical measures, to prohibit cloning for the purpose of replicating human individuals." The European Union's Council of Europe adopted the Council of Europe Protocol, prohibiting the cloning of human beings. Similarly, the European Parliament has adopted a Resolution on Human Cloning. The resolution calls for member states to enact binding national legislation banning cloning and also urges the United Nations to secure an international ban on cloning. Likewise, UNESCO's Universal Declaration on the Human Genome and Human Rights specifically addresses cloning and states, "Practices which are contrary to human dignity, such as reproductive cloning of human beings, shall not be permitted."

The Process for the Creation of an International Treaty

On August 7, 2001, France and Germany urged the U.N. secretary-general to add to the agenda for the current U.N. session an International Convention against Reproductive Cloning of Human Beings.[23] In November 2001 the Legal Committee of the United Nations added its support, and it held meetings in 2002, 2003, and 2004.

No country wants to allow use of the Dolly-the-sheep cloning technique—the one since used to create mice, pigs, cows, and, most recently, rabbits and a kitten—to make a human child. Virtually every nation agrees that children should not be commodified like barnyard animals or pets, even like beloved cats or dogs. The powerful global consensus that human reproductive cloning should be outlawed provided an unprecedented opportunity for the world to take united action on a bioethical issue that could profoundly affect the future of our species.

The United States, nonetheless, threatened to take its ball and go home if the world community did not give in to its demands to outlaw not just reproductive cloning but also research cloning. (Sometimes called "therapeutic cloning," even though no therapies have been produced, research cloning involves making human embryos by somatic cell nuclear transfer with the goal of deriving stem cells for medical research.) This all-or-nothing, take-it-or-leave-it approach is the same position taken by the House of Representatives and repeated by President George W. Bush (although not by his Council on Bioethics).

As of March 2007 the U.S. Senate has yet even to debate the ban, probably because the vote is too close to call. Nonetheless, unless a compromise can ultimately be reached so that outlawing reproductive cloning is not held hostage to banning research cloning, the likely outcome is that no law on cloning will ever pass, or if it passes, it will be vetoed by the president. Without congressional action banning reproductive cloning in the United States, the practice will likely be attempted by its radical proponents. Is there a compromise that can stop the cloning renegades while permitting legitimate medical research?

The first step toward a solution is to understand the Bush administration's position. Leon Kass, its intellectual architect and the former head of the president's Bioethics Council, has argued eloquently and passionately that if you oppose creating a child by cloning, you must also oppose creating human embryos for research by cloning. This is because, he says, if research cloning is permitted, it is inevitable that someone will try to implant one of the cloned embryos in a woman, and once this occurs, no government would ever force the woman to abort the clone. Moreover, he argues, research cloning would result in private industry stockpiling human embryos and mining, exploiting, and selling them. Opponents of research cloning have run radio ads warning of "embryo hatcheries" and "embryo farms." A ban on implanting these embryos, Kass says, would require the government to destroy cloned embryos rather than preserve and protect this form of nascent human life, an action that would be repugnant to many.

Kass reiterated this position in 2002 when he opened the first meeting of the Bioethics Council with a discussion of Nathaniel Hawthorne's "The Birthmark." In the story a scientist, Alymer, marries a beautiful young woman, Georgiana, who has a small handlike birthmark on her face. Alymer becomes obsessed with removing it, and the potion he ultimately creates to remove it also kills her. Imperfection, of course, is an inherent characteristic of humans, and attempting to make the perfect human is certainly dangerous, and ultimately impossible. Kass takes the story as a cautionary tale that science's attempt to perfect humans by, among things, changing our basic sexual nature (as by making sexual reproduction optional) could have deadly consequences.

Kass is right to caution us about the limits of our technology and the slippery slope. Alymer was wrong to see human perfection through scientific technique as a reasonable human goal, and "The Birthmark" rightly warns us about that nightmarish eugenic goal. But is the United States right to oppose research cloning aimed at finding cures for devastating human diseases and alleviating severe human suffering, historically both important and completely legitimate goals of medical research? I don't think so, at least not if we can take effective regulatory steps. And this points the way to a possible political compromise.

There are two basic ways Congress could act to stop baby-making cloners without outlawing research on cloned embryos. The first is to put a moratorium on research cloning until the use of adult stem cells is fully explored, and/or until research using stem cells from "spare" or leftover embryos created at in vitro fertilization clinics is demonstrated to be of therapeutic value in tissue regeneration. The second, and I think better and more permanent, solution is to create a regulatory framework that would make the administration's dreaded commercial stockpiles (and farms) of cloned embryos and the initiation of a pregnancy with one of them virtually impossible. This regulatory challenge is currently facing at least two states that have specifically encouraged the creation of cloned embryos for research while simultaneously outlawing replication cloning: California and Massachusetts.

Regulation is a challenge, whether on a state, federal, or worldwide basis. Historically, embryo research has never been regulated in the United States, primarily because the U.S. government has never funded it. Nonetheless, on the federal level Congress has the authority to regulate all such research, not just publicly funded research, if it wants to. In particular, Congress could greatly improve the overall ethics of now wholly unregulated research with cloned human embryos, permitting the science to proceed, and at the same time virtually guarantee that no cloned human embryo lawfully made would be implanted—or even have to be ordered destroyed by the government. Here's how it would work. Ideally, Congress would create a federal oversight authority (similar to England's Human Fertilization and Embryology Authority) that would have exclusive authority to approve any proposed embryo research project, including those in the private sector. Approval would be granted only for those projects soundly designed to address a compelling medical need that could not be successfully addressed in any other way.

To prevent the transgressions envisioned by Kass and the Bush administration, specifically the stockpiling and commercial use of cloned research embryos and the implanting of a research embryo to start a pregnancy, at least three prohibitions are required: First, the freezing and storage of cloned embryos should be outlawed. Cloned embryos would be created solely for use in approved research projects, and there is no reason to "store" or "stockpile" them because the research embryos are destroyed in the research process. A strict limit of 7 to 14 days should be placed on the length of time any cloned human embryo can be maintained. Second, and perhaps most controversial, the purchase and sale of human eggs and human embryos should be outlawed. This would help to eliminate the increasing commercialization of embryo research and the commodification of both human eggs and embryos. Finally, all individuals, including physicians, scientists, and biotech companies, who have not been approved to do research cloning must be prohibited from making or possessing cloned embryos. In addition, all in vitro fertilization clinics and physicians and embryologists associated with them would be specifically prohibited from doing research on cloned embryos, making it virtually impossible for a cloned embryo to ever be used to initiate a pregnancy.

In the absence of federal legislation, we are left to state and private initiatives. One proposal that is gaining ground is a 2005 recommendation of the Institute of Medicine to promote human embryonic stem cell research, including the use of cloning embryos, by adopting voluntary national guidelines (outlined in their report) to limit the culture of any embryo to 14 days and prohibit implantation, and also establish a "national body" to periodically review the guidelines and provide a forum for discussing them. These proposals are constructive, but to be credible any national body would have to be independent of the researchers, be well funded, and, I believe, have the authority to review and approve (or disapprove) all specific research projects involving cloned human embryos. A greater challenge, but one well worth pursuing, is to establish not only a national body but also an international body, with similar—although not government sanctioned—guideline-making authority to which both government and private entities pursing cloning research would be expected to conform. This may actually be the best hope for the immediate future.

Alymer's real crime was that he was unable to separate his love for his wife from his love of science, and in joining them, he killed her. Combining bans on both reproductive and research cloning in one bill is likely to kill the anticloning legislation as well. And because reasonable compromise is available, this lethal outcome is unnecessary. An example from another regulatory realm helps demonstrate that the law can effectively ban one activity without banning two related activities. There is a reasonable argument that an effective ban on offensive biological weapons research requires a ban on defensive biological weapons research as well. Nonetheless, it would be self-defeating and irrational to refuse to support a ban on offensive weapons research solely because defensive research was not banned simultaneously. Defensive biowarfare research can be used to make an offensive weapon, of course, but this requires both a much greater volume of toxins as well as their introduction into a delivery system. Likewise, cloned embryos could be used to make babies, but we are much more likely to prevent this eventuality with a ban on implanting human cloned embryos coupled with regulation of embryo research than with no regulation of cloning at all. We can outlaw cloning to create children without outlawing cloning to create medicines.

International Gridlock

Actions of the U.S. Senate and the United Nations are a moving target. Nonetheless, in 2005 the United States persuaded the world that it could effectively block a treaty that did not outlaw research cloning, and as a consequence the United Nations agreed in early 2005 to promulgate a Declaration (which is a statement of aspirations rather than a legally binding instrument) on human cloning. The language of the United Nations Declaration on Human Cloning is as follows (and can be usefully contrasted to the treaty proposal quoted at the beginning of this chapter):

> *Guided* by the purposes and principles of the Charter of the United Nations,

Recalling the Universal Declaration on the Human Genome and Human Rights . . .

Aware of the ethical concerns that certain applications of rapidly developing life sciences may raise with regard to human dignity, human rights and the fundamental freedoms of individuals,

Reaffirming that the application of life sciences should seek to offer relief from suffering and improve the health of individual and humankind as a whole,

Emphasizing that the promotion of scientific and technical progress in life sciences should be sought in a manner that safeguards respect for human rights and the benefit of all,

Mindful of the serious medical, physical, psychological and social dangers that human cloning may imply for the individuals involved, and also conscious of the need to prevent the exploitation of women,

Convinced of the urgency of preventing the potential dangers of human cloning to human dignity,

Solemnly declares the following:

(a) Member States are called on to adopt all measures necessary to protect adequately human life in the application of the life sciences;

(b) Member States are called on to prohibit all forms of human cloning inasmuch as they are incompatible with human dignity and the protection of human life;

(c) Member States are further called on to adopt the measures necessary to prohibit the application of genetic engineering techniques that may be contrary to human dignity;

(d) Member States are called on to take measures to prevent the exploitation of women in the application of life sciences;

(e) Member States are also called on to adopt and implement without delay national legislation to bring into effect paragraphs (a) to (d);

(f) Member States are further called on, in their financing of medical research, including of life sciences, to take into account the pressing global issues such as HIV/AIDS, tuberculosis and malaria, which affect in particular the developing countries.[24]

Unfortunately, these statements are vague enough to permit each individual country to do what it thinks is right; by its own terms, a Declaration does not require a country to take any action at all. In short, the United Nations' attempt to set up a regulatory scheme to outlaw human reproductive cloning has been halted for the immediate future. With the cloning logjam, it may make more political sense to concentrate exclusively on a treaty on the real species-endangering activity, inheritable genetic alteration, because there is no support for this activity by any government or scientific organization in the world. Simultaneously, private efforts to set up a global voluntary oversight body should be vigorously pursued. The first small steps toward this goal have been taken by the private International Society for Stem Cell Research, which promulgated its initial "Guidelines for Human Embryonic Stem Cell Research" in early 2007.[25] These are a beginning.

Conclusion

Biotechnology, especially human cloning and germline genetic engineering, have the potential to permit us to design our children and literally to change the characteristics of the human species. The movement toward a posthuman world can be characterized as progress and an enhancement of individual freedom in the area of procreation, but it also can be characterized as a movement down a slippery slope to a neoeugenics that will result in the creation of one or more subspecies or superspecies of humans. The first vision sees science as our guide and ultimate goal. The second is more firmly based on our human history, which has consistently emphasized differences and has used those differences to justify genocidal actions. It is the prospect of "genetic genocide" that calls for treating cloning and genetic engineering as potential weapons of mass destruction and the unaccountable genetic researcher as a potential bioterrorist.

The greatest accomplishment of humans has not been our science but our development of human rights and democracy. Science deals with facts, not values. It cannot, for example, tell us whether immortality, even limited to genetic immortality, is good for either individuals or the human species. Because science cannot tell us what we should do, or even what our goals are, humans must give direction to science. In the area of genetics, this calls for international action to control the techniques that could lead us to commit species suicide. We humans recognized the risk clearly in splitting the atom and developing nuclear weapons, and most humans recognize the risk in using human genes to modify ourselves. Because the risk is to the entire species, it requires a species response. Many countries have already enacted bans, moratoria, and strict regulations on various species-altering technologies. The challenge, however, remains global, and action on the international level is required to be effective.

One action called for today is the ratification of an international Convention for the Preservation of the Human Species that outlaws human cloning and inheritable genetic alterations, or at least the latter. This ban would not only be important for itself but would also mark the first time the world worked together to control a biotechnology. Cloning and inheritable genetic modifications are not bioweapons per se, but they could prove just as destructive to the human species if left to the market and to individual wants and desires. An international consensus to ban these technologies already exists, and countries, NGOs, and individual citizens should actively support a renewed treaty process, as they did with the recent Convention on the Prohibition of the Use, Stockpiling, Production and Transfer of Anti-personnol Mines and their Destruction (Mine Ban Treaty).

Inheritable genetic alteration of children may not seem as important as land mines because no child with such an attempted alteration has yet been born and thus no child has yet been harmed by this technique. Nonetheless, the use of inheritable genetic alteration (and human replicative cloning) has the potential to harm all children, both directly by limiting the genetically modified children's freedom and harming them physically and mentally, and indirectly by devaluing all children by treating them as products of their parents' genetic specifications. Of more concern, inheritable genetic alteration carries the prospect of developing a new species or subspecies of humans, who could turn into either destroyers or victims of the human species. Opposition to cloning and inheritable genetic alteration is conservative in the strict sense of the word: it seeks to conserve the human species. But it is also liberal in the strict sense of the word: it seeks to preserve democracy, freedom, and universal human rights for all members of the human species.

Proponents of going full speed ahead with inheritable genetic alterations are fond of quoting Thucydides in his *History of the Peloponnesian War* to the effect that "the bravest are surely those with the clearest vision of the future, disaster and benefit alike, and that not withstanding these possibilities they move ahead" (1954, 147). Sounds great, but when placed in historical context, the statement actually supports application of the precautionary principle to inheritable genetic alterations. The statement is made by the great Athenian general, Pericles, in his famous funeral ora-tion praising the nature of Athenian citizenship. His real point is not that Athenians are impulsive and brave as a character trait, but rather that as a democracy they think before they act and weigh the possible consequences before voting on how to proceed. As Pericles puts it concisely, "The worst thing is to rush into action before the consequences have been properly debated." And later, when Athens is in the midst of a disastrous war, Thucydides, a former general himself, describes how war changes what we think of as virtue: "What used to be described as a thoughtless act of aggression was now regarded as courage . . . to think of the future and wait was merely another way of saying one was a coward . . . ability to understand a question from all sides meant that one was totally unfitted for action. Fanatical enthusiasm was the mark of a real man" (242).

Whether in private laboratories and corporations or on the state, federal, or global level, the ethical and human rights challenge remains to protect the human rights of children by prohibiting their genetic manufacture while permitting legitimate research designed to make new medicines to proceed. We can, in short, pursue regenerative medicine without simultaneously pursuing replicative medicine, seeking immortality, or producing the posthuman.

NOTES

1. Major portions of this chapter are adapted from Annas, Andrews, and Isasi (2002), which contains more detailed notes and references, and Annas (2002), both of which were the basis of chapter 4 of *American Bioethics: Crossing Human Rights and Health Law Boundaries* (New York: Oxford University Press, 2005). The material in these sources has been updated to March 1, 2007.

2. See, for example, Fukuyama, 2002. And see note 14.

3. See, for example, Raffensperger and Tickner, 1999.

4. This proposed Convention is the product of many people, including the participants at a September 21–22, 2001, conference at Boston University entitled "Beyond Cloning: Protecting Humanity from Species-Altering Procedures." The treaty language was the subject of a roundtable that concluded the conference. The authors, together with others, most especially Patricia Baird and Alexander Capron, had drafted language to be considered at the conference and revised it after the conference based on the discussion that occurred there. The original draft also included a codicil to encourage individual countries to examine broader issues related to the regulation of assisted human reproduction and a prohibition on the patenting of human genes.

5. See also National Bioethics Advisory Commission, 1997, as well as President's Council on Bioethics, 2002, which recommends banning human reproductive cloning and placing a time-limited moratorium on research cloning.

6. National Research Council, 2002: "Human reproductive cloning . . . is dangerous and likely to fail. The panel therefore unanimously supports the proposal that there should be a legally enforceable ban on the practice of human reproductive cloning . . . The scientific and medical considerations related to this ban should be reviewed within 5 years. The ban should be reconsidered only if at least two conditions are met: (1) a new scientific and medical review indicates that the procedures are likely to be safe and effective and (2) a broad national dialogue on the societal, religious, and ethical issues suggests that a reconsideration of the ban is warranted" (ES–1). See also National Research Council, 2001, and Jaenisch and Wilmut, 2001: "We believe attempts to clone human beings at a time when the scientific issues of nuclear cloning have not be clarified are dangerous and irresponsible."

7. Stuart A. Newman, oral presentation at the "Beyond Cloning " conference, Boston University, Boston, September 21, 2001. Other scientists have concluded that nuclear transfer cloning in primates, including humans, is simply "unachievable" with "current approaches" (Simerly, 2003).

8. See, for example, Gordon, 1999.

9. Hans Jonas, for example, argued that it is a crime against the clone in that it deprives the cloned child of his or her "existential right to certain subjective terms of being . . . the right to ignorance [of facts about the original that are likely to be] paralyzing for the spontaneity of becoming himself . . . in brief, the clone is antecedently robbed of the freedom which only under the protection of ignorance can thrive: and to rob a human-to-be of that freedom deliberately is an inexplicable crime that must not be committed even once" (Jonas, 1974, 162–63).

10. Adams, 2001. See also Winston, 1997 (arguing in favor of using cloning to help infertile men have genetically related children).

11. See, generally, Shapiro, 1999.

12. For example, American Society of Reproductive Medicine, Ethics Committee, Human Somatic Cell Nuclear Transfer (cloning), November 2000, www.asrm.org/Media/Ethics/cloning.pdf.

13. See, generally, Hall, 2003.

14. For an excellent summary of the arguments on both sides of the genetic enhancement debate, see Garreau, 2005. Related specifically to immortality, Garreau quotes Francis Fukuyama as saying about possible immortality both that it would mean the end of innovation—in that the immortals would be incapable of having a new idea—and, more important, as asking, "Can [immortals] conceive of dying for a cause higher than themselves and their own fucking little petty lives?" (163).

15. Rosario Isasi compiled all of the national legislation related to cloning and human genetic engineering. It appears on the Global Lawyers and Physicians website, www.glphr.org.

16. See Annas and Grodin, 1992.

17. It is in this sense that children become "manufactured" products. See Kass, 1985.

18. See Fukuyama, 2002, and Mehlman, 2003, 100–91. But see Stock and Campbell, 2000, and Garreau, 2005, for arguments favoring the use of inheritable genetic alterations.

19. See, for example, the post-Dolly experiments designed to use cloning techniques to make "better animals," which was always Ian Wilmut and Keith Campbell's plan for cloning technology (Shnieke et al., 1997). On enhancement generally, see Rothman and Rothman, 2003.

20. See Kress's Beggars series, *Beggars in Spain* (1993), *Beggars and Choosers* (1994), and *Beggars Ride* (1996).

21. See notes 1 and 15 for details regarding these laws.

22. "Regulatory arbitrage" is a fancy term for seeking overseas venues to avoid local research regulations. One such venue is South Korea, which has the current world lead in human research cloning. On the other hand, most scientists seem to want to work in their own countries, and although the Korean cloners initially threatened to leave South Korea to pursue their work, they almost immediately agreed to work under new governmental regulations (Faiola, 2004). See, generally, Isasi and Annas, 2003.

23. Document A/56/192 of 7 August 2001, Request for the inclusion of a supplementary item in the agenda of the fifty-sixth session, International Convention against the Reproductive Cloning of Human Beings, available at www.un.org/ga/56/document.htm.

24. 59/280, United Nations Declaration on Human Cloning. It is well worth noting that although a majority of countries voting voted in favor of this declaration (46% of the total number of countries), on a population basis, countries voting in favor represented 1.5 billion people; not voting, 1.6 billion (36% of all countries that abstained or were absent); and voting against, 3.1 billion (18% of all countries). The message is that most people want to (and will) pursue research cloning, including the world's most populous countries, China and India. See also Annas, 2005, and Isasi and Annas, 2006.

25. See Daley, 2007. Currently, the most controversial issue both nationally and internationally is the question of payment to women for their ova for use in research cloning. This issue has prompted increased attention to the question of risk to the ova donors. See, for example, Committee on Assessing the Medical Risks of Human Oocyte Donation for Stem Cell Research, 2007.

REFERENCES

Adams, T. 2001. Interview: The clone arranger. *The Observer (London),* December 2.

Annas, G. J. 2002. Cell division. *Boston Globe,* April 21, D1.

Annas, G. J. 2005. The ABCs of global governance of embryonic stem cell research: Arbitrage, bioethics, and cloning. *New England Law Review* 39:489–500.

Annas, G. J., and M. A. Grodin, eds. 1992. *The Nazi Doctors and the Nuremberg Code.* New York: Oxford University Press.

Bassiouni, M. Cherif. 1992. *Crimes against Humanity in International Criminal Law.* Dordrecht: Martinus Nijhoff.

Committee on Assessing the Medical Risks of Human Oocyte Donation for Stem Cell Research. 2007. *Assessing the Medical Risks of Human Oocyte Donation for Stem Cell Research: Workshop Report.* Washington, DC: National Academies Press.

Daley, G. Q., et al. 2007. The ISSCR guidelines for human embryonic stem cell research. *Science* 315:603–4.

Dworkin, R. 2000. *Sovereign Virtue: The Theory and Practice of Equality.* Cambridge, MA: Harvard University Press.

Faiola, A. 2004. Dr. Clone. *Washington Post,* February 29.

Fukuyama, F. 2002. *Our Posthuman Future.* New York: Farrar, Straus and Giroux.

Garreau, J. 2005. *Radical Evolution: The Promise and Peril of Enhancing Our Minds, Our Bodies—and What It Means to Be Human.* New York: Doubleday.

Gordon, J. W. 1999. Genetic enhancement in humans. *Science* 283:202–3.

Hall, S. S. 2003. *Merchants of Immortality.* New York: Houghton Mifflin.

Institute of Medicine. 2005. *Guidelines for Human Embryonic Stem Cell Research,* April 26.

Isasi, R. M., and G. J. Annas. 2003. Arbitrage, bioethics, and cloning: The ABCs of gestating a United Nations cloning convention. *Case Western Reserve Journal of International Law* 35:397–414.

Isasi, R. M., and G. J. Annas. 2006. To clone alone: The United Nations' human cloning declaration. *Law and the Human Genome Review* 24:13–26.

Jaenisch, R., and I. Wilmut. 2001. Don't clone humans! *Science* 291:2552.

Jonas, H. 1974. *Philosophical Essays: From Ancient Creed to Technological Man.* New York: Prentice-Hall.

Kass, L. R. 1985. *Toward a More Natural Science: Biology and Human Affairs.* New York: Free Press.

Kress, N. 1993. *Beggars in Spain.* New York: William Morrow.

Kress, N. 1994. *Beggars and Choosers.* New York: TOR.

Kress, N. 1996. *Beggars Ride.* New York: TOR.

Mehlman, M. J. 2003. *Wondergenes.* Bloomington: University of Indiana Press.

National Bioethics Advisory Commission. 1997. *Cloning Human Beings.* Bethesda, MD: The Commission.

National Research Council. 2001. *Stem Cells and the Future of Regenerative Medicine.* Washington, DC: National Academy Press.

National Research Council. 2002. *Scientific and Medical Aspects of Human Reproductive Cloning.* Washington, DC: National Academy Press.

Nature. 2007. Editorial: Dolly's legacy. *Nature* 445:795.

Pinker, S. 2003. Better babies? Why genetic enhancement is too unlikely to worry about. *Boston Globe,* June 1, D1.

President's Council on Bioethics. 2002. *Human Cloning and Human Dignity.* New York: Public Affairs.

Rael. 1998. *The True Face of God.* Geneva: International Raelian Movement.

Raffensperger, C., and J. A. Tickner, eds. 1999. *Protecting Public Health and the Environment: Implementing the Precautionary Principle.* Washington, DC: Island Press.

Robertson, J. 1999. Two models of human cloning. *Hofstra Law Review* 27:609.

Rothman, S., and D. Rothman. 2003. *The Pursuit of Perfection.* New York: Pantheon Books.

Shapiro, M. H. 1999. I want a girl (boy) just like the girl (boy) that married dear old Dad (Mom): Cloning lives. *Southern California Interdisciplinary Law Journal* 9:1.

Shnieke, A. E., et al. 1997. Human factor IX transgenic sheep produced by transfer of nuclei from transplanted fetal fibroblasts. *Science* 278:2130.

Silver, L. 1997. *Remaking Eden: Cloning and Beyond in a Brave New World.* New York: Avon Books.

Simerly, C., et al. 2003. Molecular correlates of primate nuclear failures. *Science* 300:297.

Stock, G., and J. Campbell, eds. 2000. *Engineering the Human Germline.* New York: Oxford University Press.

Thucydides. 1954. *History of the Peloponnesian War,* trans. Rex. Warner. London: Penguin Books.

Winston, R. 1997. The promise of cloning for human medicine. *British Medical Journal* 314:913–14.

CHAPTER 4

The Transhumanist Movement

A Flawed Response to Aging and Its Natural Consequence

THOMAS A. SHANNON, PH.D.

To speak of the posthuman or the transhuman suggests a prehuman and a human that preceded the posthuman. If one buys into evolution, as approximately 53 percent of Americans do, the prehuman comes from the various life forms that preceded us and formed our immediate ancestors. The human emerged, taking some first tenuous steps out of Africa and then rather quickly moving around the world and settling in all the continents and began increasing and multiplying. This, then, brings us to the posthuman or transhuman.

A problem seems to be that just as in the transition from prehuman to human, there was a lot of overlap and coexistence with the prehuman and human, so too there is apparently a lot of overlap between the human and the posthuman. Some, I suspect, do not even know that there are such beings as posthumans or transhumans. Such people, of course, do not live on college campuses, where all three types seem to exist in various stages of appearance and in a variety of relationships.

The critical difference between the transition from prehuman to human and human to posthuman is that in the former the mechanism of transition was primarily natural selection augmented by various environmental factors, such as climate, food supply, and natural disasters of one type or another. The process of evolution was at work, and selections occurred. In our current situation, evolution continues to occur, though because of the time the process takes, we tend not to be significantly aware of it, just as we are not aware of the movement of the tectonic plates under our feet ever so slowly causing the rearrangement of the earth's surface.

But in addition to the gradual and steady work of evolution, there is another process important to consider as we think of the posthuman. This other process is culture. While the reality of culture is probably coeval with the emergence of at least modern *Homo sapiens,* it is clearly present with us and exerts a force on our evolutionary directions. While biological evolution moves along through the impersonal process of natural selection, culture influences evolution by setting out goals, desires, and values. And while at some level, cultural evolution may be also impersonal, it gives the opportunity to influence evolution, to attempt to override or to reject biology and natural selection altogether. For example, the standard ratio of male to female births among humans is about 105 to 100, but within a few years the ratio balances out to about 100 to 100, owing to a higher rate of male infant mortality. In the Fujian Province of China, however, the birth ratio is 134 males for every 100 females. There are two reasons for this skewed ratio, both cultural: one is the value of the male child as the primary form of social security for the parents, particularly in rural areas, and the second is the one-child-per-family policy implemented to help decrease the population. Given the first reason, if you are supposed to have only one child, that child had better be a male. The various technologies of prenatal diagnosis combined with selective abortion make that choice a reality. Individual choices have social consequences, and demographers estimate that within a few decades, there could be as many as 40 million men unable to find mates. The solutions to this problem are equally culture- and technology-dependent: cash and educational subsidies for female infants (Yardley, 2005). Culture and evolution collided and culture won, but the victory came at a price.

The search for the posthuman manifests a tension between the process of evolution and the process of culture. This is not a debate between determinism and freedom but a negotiation between some biological phenomena and some cultural realities. The discussion needs to be cast this way because we humans are as much our biology as we are our culture. We are somatic as well as transcendent. We are animated flesh.

From the biological perspective, there are some realities to be observed. First, we are contingent beings. There is no necessary line from the first organism emerging out of the primal slime eons ago to us. That we are here as opposed to other species of *Homo* that also were evolving is a function of natural selection and reproductive success. And in the later stages of evolution, culture also complimented what was occurring biologically. Second, we are here, but evolution continues. Though its pace is slow and almost imperceptible, evolution is a continuing process. As long as there is life, there will be evolution, and the consequence of that is change—descent with modification. We are thus a work in process, not a finished product by any stretch of the imagination. Third, because we are in process, who or what our species will become—or even whether it will survive—is an open question. Species come and species go, and in between they do not stay the same. Fourth, we are not the crown of creation. We are one branch among other branches. Our DNA is the DNA of all other living organisms, and what future expressions of this DNA will be remains to be seen. Fifth, diversity is the consequence of evolution, and the primary mechanism of diversity is sexual recombination. This recombination helps shape the fitness of an organism for survival but also provides the genetic basis for the capacity to adapt to a variety of changing environments. The more diverse an organism is, the more robust it is with respect to survival. Finally, species and the individuals within them are finite, that is, they die. If they did not die, there would be no room for the ones coming along. Death is a survival mechanism for life. It allows newness and diversity to take root and flourish and diversify. This last reality is a particularly hard one personally, socially, and culturally, but death is a most critical mechanism of change.

Yet we are also deeply creatures of culture. As we have evolved, we have produced institutions, mores, practices, values, religions, civilizations. We have generated systems of meaning, a sense of the transcendent, a taste for a future, the desire for the new or the different. In short, we might even argue that fundamentally what culture gives us is desire, a desire that transcends the biological. And this cultural dimension of ourselves and our species is powerful. For the sake of some cultural ideals, individuals will renounce sexual activity, will put their lives in mortal danger, will delay gratification of needs for decades, and will seek to transform or alter their very biology.

A culture also gives each of us a starting point, some sense of givens as we attempt to wend our way through our life and the lives of those around us. Though we are born with some instincts and with a biology that operates on its own, that is not enough for human survival. Our evolutionary path has taken us beyond day-to-day survival to the gifts of culture so that we may plan ahead, make provision for the future, and seek a good life. Clearly these values and cultural starting points—science, technology, education, politics, religion, family—change over time as they and we seek to adapt to the new, but they also provide a sense of continuity and stability as we move through society.

As we begin to think of ourselves, these biological and cultural realities form a context in which we must think and evaluate and plan. I do not understand how it is possible to consider ourselves, our nature, and our future without incorporating some of the reality of these evolutionary and cultural structures that have brought us to our current location.

The Transhumanist and Posthumanist Culture

The transhumanist movement provides an interesting case study on the meaning of human nature and its limits. This movement has its origins in part in the human regeneration movement. The early origins of the movement were the traditional European spas but also the Clinique La Prairie, in Clarens, Switzerland, operated by Dr. Paul Niehans. The primary treatment was the injection of fetal sheep cells into humans. Of concern to the movement is the tragedy that our bodies and our death bring into human life: "Modern transhumanism is a statement of disappointment. Transhumans regard our bodies as sadly inadequate, limited by our physiognomy, which restricts our brain power, our strength, and, the world of all our lifespan" (Alexander, 2003, 51).

This perspective answers with a resounding no the primal question emerging from Samuel Becket's plays: "Is personal extinction worth the wait?" (Isherwoon, 2005, B2). The transhumanist disappointment with personal extinction and the "powerful vision of life as a game stacked against us all" (Isherwoon, 2005 B2) of necessity looks for solutions, not in the traditional places, but in improvements that will come from technol-

ogy, bioengineering, and genetics, with some nods to cryonics. An acro-
nym for the movement was coined by Timothy Leary after his "turn-on,
tune in, and drop out" phase (Alexander, 2003, 54): SMILE, for Space Mi-
gration, I^2 (the doubling of human intelligence), and Life Extension. And
there was a countertype (Alexander, 2003, 59): MOSH, Mostly Original
Substrate Humans. And by means of computer jacks inserted in one's head,
one could live in a world of virtual reality and become who one wished
whenever one wished. Such a vision is summarized by Ray Kurzweil (2002,
51), who said, "Ultimately software-based humans, albeit vastly extended
beyond the severe limitations of humans as we know them today, will live
out on the web, projecting bodies whenever they need or want them, including virtual bodies in diverse realms of virtual reality, holographically
projected bodies and physical bodies comprised of nanobot swarms, and
other forms of nanotechnology."

The Principles of Extropy in Brief

Eventually a Declaration of Extropian Principles was generated. Extropy
was the contrary of entropy and signaled the constant improvement of
humans to the point where they became an entirely new species, in part
through the assistance of various nanotechnologies that would solve most
of our problems. More (2003) outlined the basic principles of extropy as
follows:

> *Perpetual Progress.* Extropy means seeking more intelligence, wisdom,
> and effectiveness, an open-ended lifespan, and the removal of political,
> cultural, biological, and psychological limits to continuing development.
> Perpetually overcoming constraints on our progress and possibilities as
> individuals, as organizations, and as a species. Growing in healthy
> directions without bound.
>
> *Self-Transformation.* Extropy means affirming continual ethical,
> intellectual, and physical self-improvement, through critical and creative
> thinking, perpetual learning, personal responsibility, proactivity, and
> experimentation. Using technology—in the widest sense to seek physi-
> ological and neurological augmentation along with emotional and psycho-
> logical refinement.
>
> *Practical Optimism.* Extropy means fueling action with positive
> expectations, individuals and organizations being tirelessly proactive.

Adopting a rational, action-based optimism or "proaction," in place of both blind faith and stagnant pessimism.

Intelligent Technology. Extropy means designing and managing technologies not as ends in themselves but as effective means for improving life. Applying science and technology creatively and courageously to transcend "natural" but harmful, confining qualities derived from our biological heritage, culture, and environment.

Open Society. Extropy means supporting social orders that foster freedom of communication, freedom of action, experimentation, innovation, questioning, and learning. Opposing authoritarian social control and unnecessary hierarchy and favoring the rule of law and decentralization of power and responsibility. Preferring bargaining over battling, exchange over extortion, and communication over compulsion. Openness to improvement rather than a static utopia. Extropia ("ever-receding stretch goals for society") over utopia ("no place").

Self-Direction. Extropy means valuing independent thinking, individual freedom, personal responsibility, self-direction, self-respect, and a parallel respect for others.

Rational Thinking. Extropy means favoring reason over blind faith and questioning over dogma. It means understanding, experimenting, learning, challenging, and innovating rather than clinging to beliefs.

As one reads these, it is hard not to agree with many of the sentiments expressed. Who does not value at least some degree of rationality, negotiation rather than battles, freedom and responsibility? Yet underneath the surface and sometimes on the surface, the transhumanist discontent with the status quo, the rejection of limits, and the affirmation of growth without bounds emerge as salient features. A deep restlessness with the status quo and the way things are is the underlying motive to move us to our new transhuman future. And according to some in the movement, "The future belonged to molecular biology, which had the power to salve human desperation over disease and death" (More, 2003, 79). Death was simply not to be accepted. Or, as phrased by Robert Edwards, of IVF fame in England, "We are the last five minutes of evolution and we have gone wrong! Badly wrong!" (More, 2003, 149).

As I have noted, a variety of means have been proposed to eliminate the problem of death: supplements, diets, exercise, computers, biotechnology, cryogenics, and possibly cloning. Additionally a great deal of sexual activity with many partners seems to be part of the equation, if one is to believe the sometimes breathless prose in *The Rapture* (Alexander, 2003), a book that highlights many of the activities of a select group of self-proclaimed posthumans. One also seems to need a fair amount of money to purchase the required supplies, to have the leisure time to pursue these activities, and to travel to all the centers and conferences. Nancie Clark, who changed her name to Natasha Vita-More to express her desire for more life, has a demanding workout schedule (Vita-More, 1997) that combines anaerobic exercise (bodybuilding) and aerobic sports (downhill skiing and cycling). Ray Kurzweil reportedly takes "250 supplements, eight to 10 glasses of alkaline water and 10 cups of green tea. He also periodically tracks 40 to 50 fitness indicators, down to his 'tactile sensitivity.' Adjustments are made as needed" (Linsay, 2005).

Additionally there are several goals to which one should aspire as the consequence of this dedication to physical fitness, to a transformed body, to a new self (Vita-More, 2005). Helpfully, a comparison list is provided:

Twentieth Century: Body	Twenty-first Century: Primo Posthuman
Limited life span	Ageless
Legacy genes	Replaceable genes
Wears out	Upgrades
Random mistakes	Error correction device
Sense of humanity	Enlightened transhumanity
Intelligence capacity 100 trillion synapses	Intelligence capacity 100 quadrillion synapses
Single track awareness	Multiple viewpoints running in parallel
Gender restricted	Gender changeability
Prone to environmental damage	Impervious to environmental damage
Corrosion by irritability, envy, depression	Turbocharged optimism
Elimination of messy and gaseous waste	Recycles and purifies waste

What is interesting in this is the utter flexibility of the transhuman, including upgraded genes, gender variability, and heightened intelligence. Also interesting is that the design is impervious to environmental damage. Thus, should those not at the transhuman stage continue to muck up the environment, the transhumans need not worry. And how is such a movement to be started? Typically there is a revolutionary vanguard, and the transhumans are no different. The "Supercentenarian Research Foundation" website (www.mprize.org/index.php?pagename=thethreehundred) begins with the following: "What's it worth to you to live 150 healthy years? What's it worth to you to raise the average human lifespan to 150 years, just as a start? These are not idle questions! Membership of The Three Hundred is a meaningful, but affordable commitment: $1,000 a year, by the end of each year, for 25 years. This amounts to $85 a month or $2.75 a day, the equivalent of a visit to Starbucks."

The text continues with a discussion of "The Three Hundred":

We call it "The Three Hundred" . . . themed from history and limited to that number of participants. These individuals (or organizations) see the potential of the Prize and believe that aging can be defeated. Members of The Three Hundred have made a commitment to creating a better future, one in which the suffering caused by aging is greatly diminished or banished entirely. The unique foresight shared by The Three Hundred at this early stage in aging research will be remembered—they grasped the ring, heard the call and took action when the opportunity first presented itself. The efforts of the Three Hundred will be remembered, like those of their historical counterparts, far into the future.

The Three Hundred is a classical concept, based on a battle that saved the future of Western Civilization: Thermopylae. In 480 B.C., 300 Spartan warriors fought against incredible odds to gain time for the rest of Greece to mobilize against the Persian hordes. Without the delaying action fought at the narrow pass of Thermopylae, the achievements of Greece and our culture as we know it would have been swept away.

The Methuselah Foundation is asking you to follow in the footsteps of this noble Three Hundred, not to risk your lives, but to provide some of your treasure so that we can all live . . . and live . . . and live. You will help to win time for the human species to beat back an enemy far more dangerous than the ancient Persians: the Grim Reaper himself.

The Three Hundred—a group strictly limited to 300 members—will live on in history, as the Three Hundred of Thermopylae are remembered even to this day. You can be one of them. The names of the 300 Spartans who fought at Thermopylae were engraved on a stone tablet in Sparta that was still legible seven centuries later. A monument stands to this day to pay homage to their sacrifice. In lending your name to this enterprise, you will be remembered for as long as the human race survives.

The existence of The Three Hundred resonates with those who feel the injustice of the aging process, people who welcome the first serious attempts in human history to fight aging and win. Nine enthusiastic individuals have signed up before we could even make the announcement public.

Evaluation of the Transhumanist and Posthumanist Movement
General Cultural Resonance

One of the issues that has struck me as I have read some of the transhumanist literature and learned about some of these individuals is how somewhat traditional this all sounds. After all, they are talking about something that seems almost endemic to human life: enhancement. For example, if there is any common denominator to parenthood, it is surely the desire to pass on a better life to one's children. Whatever the situation of the parents, one of their fondest hopes seems to be a better legacy for their offspring—and perhaps even for their grandchildren.

Part of this desire in the United States is related to the dream of our immigrant ancestors who came here for a better life for them and their children. These immigrants arrived with little, worked hard, sacrificed, saved, and eventually made a better life for their children. They got them assimilated into the American culture, put them in private elementary and secondary schools, and then got them to attend college. The American dream was, and continues to be, realized in the enhanced lives of many immigrants.

Part of this desire is also a function of the competitive spirit that lies deep within our culture. American culture encourages winning and whatever is necessary to win, whether this be the proper networking, the right college, the right social circle, the right clothes, the right donations to worthy causes. All of these efforts are social enhancements calculated to gain the competitive edge.

Another element of enhancement in our culture is all the self-help movements, the 12-step programs, all manner of therapeutic practices, all the spa treatments. These focus on discovering and releasing the powers within the self so that one can live life better and more fully.

The cosmetic industry—whether pharmaceutical or surgical—is devoted to enhancement. This point is too obvious to comment on further.

There is also a religious dimension to enhancement in that we are continually exhorted to be better, to be transformed, and to seek perfection. In some ways we can think of penitential practices and seasons such as Lent as enhancement practices in that they are to help us transform ourselves into better practitioners of our religion and better persons. Religious life is a journey of ever-increasing perfection.

Enhancement is part and parcel of our daily lives even though we may not have thought of it in that way. Every time we use the word *better,* we are speaking enhancement language regardless of whether this refers to a car, a house, a dishwasher, clothes, or our life partner or a child. Job reviews are standard mechanisms of enhancement in that we are to specify new goals that will better our performance. Grading of students by faculty is to enhance performance on the next assignment. Our lives are lived in an atmosphere of enhancement.[1]

Death and Immortality

Another item that struck me in the transhumanist literature is the desire to eliminate death. Death as an insult to humans is a common theme of many transhumans. But I have two reflections on this. First, death is one of the major means by which change occurs. If individual and species did not in fact die out, then life would stagnate; we would in fact run out of room because no one would ever leave the room; all life would always be as it is. Species die out both so that new species can arise and so as to make room for these new ones. Thus, in many ways the transhumanist movement is profoundly antievolution. Many do, to be fair, speak of our evolving beyond the carbon-based entities we currently are, but the goal is to live forever, to eliminate the termination of my life.

The second issue that strikes me is that the affirmation of immortality is central to many religions. Most of the religions that affirm immortality also affirm some sort of dualistic anthropology in which the spirit lives on after bodily death, but others affirm a resurrection of the body and some sort of reunion of body and spirit. Important to note in this is that the resurrected and transformed being is the same being as before. There is, as some forms of Christianity proclaim, a new heaven and a new earth, but this new heaven and earth are populated by the inhabitants of the old earth, though in a transformed way, living in the new city of Jerusalem where there will be no more weeping and no more tears.

One might think that there might be some congruence here. To some degree there is with the general enhancement movement. But the transhumanist movement, while clearly looking for enhancement, also transcends it by radically redefining humans and moving to a new species altogether. Thus, in the desire to transcend, humans as we know them are left behind. But such a position also coheres somewhat with the movement of evolution: descent through modification. After all, all of our ancestors have been transcended through the evolutionary process, which is precisely how we got here. But we can trace our ancestry back to them. Though we are different, we are different only in our configuration of the same DNA that we share with them. Yet that DNA is restructured and reorganized to result in our current species of modern humans. And clearly we are still evolving, though the timeframe of evolution makes it difficult to perceive that. The critical difference is the means of evolution: DNA versus nanotechnologies that will move us from our carbon-based forms to virtual realities existing in the Internet, but with the goal of preserving the same patterns of energy so that we will survive. Thus, the technological evolution is ironically dedicated to maintaining core elements of the status quo: my existence. Life will change, but I will remain.

Responses
Philosophical Responses

The problem with the transhumanist movement, ultimately, is both its sense of disappointment at life as it is and its sense that evolution has gone badly. Here there is a profound despair, lack of trust, a denial of finitude, and an inability to accept any fate other than the one chosen by the new transhumans. Death is thus the ultimate insult to the human and the primary obstacle to be overcome. Eternal life through bioengineering and nanotechnology is the hope. Thus, Kurzweil wants to live long enough to live forever, "a seismic development he predicts in his new book is no more than 20 years away" (Linsay, 2005).

Yet life as we know it is contingent and finite. That seems to be its essence. We begin at a particular time, we exist within a variety of limits, and we die. One response to this is philosophical. One strand of the response can be found in the Heidegerian description of the human as a "Sein zur Tode," a being unto death. This perspective frankly acknowledges the reality of death and that life is a journey to that end. But this does not result in pessimism. Rather, it contains the mandate to seize the opportunity presented to us in the moment, to live each moment as if it were our last. We live our journey to death by living each moment to the fullest.

Another strand of the response to this comes from Albert Camus in his essay "The Myth of Sisyphus." Sisyphus is condemned to pushing a rock to the top of a hill. Each time he reaches the summit, however, the rock rolls back to the bottom, and Sisyphus must return to the bottom and begin again. Though many would find this an exercise in total futility, Camus argues that Sisyphus finds meaning and even some comfort in the task. Sisyphus becomes conscious of his fate, accepts it, and thus transcends it. Camus (1955, 51) argues that in the acknowledgment of one's fate, joy begins to emerge: "In the universe suddenly restored to its silence, the myriad wondering little voices of the earth rise up. Unconscious, secret calls, invitations fill the faces, they are the necessary reverse and price of victory. There is no sun without shadow, and it is essential to know the night. The absurd man says yes and his effort will henceforth be unceasing . . . The struggle itself toward the heights is enough to fill a man's heart."

One can also look to the distinction between being and having drawn so eloquently by Gabriel Marcel, one of the French existentialists. Marcel (1965, 164) notes that "having as such seems to have a tendency to destroy and lose itself in the very thing it began by possessing, but which now absorbs the master who thought he controlled it. It seems that is of the very nature of my body, or of my instruments in so far as I treat them as possessions, that they should tend to blot me out, although it is I who possess them." This observation is interesting in light of the intense efforts that many transhumanists seem to make to grasp their lives and various capacities. Marcel notes a little further on: "Our possessions eat us up" (165). My sense is that the intense fixation that this movement seems to have on the possession of life and a certain lifestyle may go very badly. The emphasis on possessing, developing, or enhancing what one has may simply end up consuming the lives of these individuals, and their reality will in fact narrow instead of expanding and prospering. Elements of the transhumanist lifestyle seem to focus narrowly on the self and thus result in a constricted vision of life, one ironically focused on the limits of the very body they are seeking to transcend.

Thus, one needs to turn to being rather than having. If we perceive our body as yet another possession, we will be alienated from it. It will no longer be animated flesh, our modality of presence in the world, but an object, a thing of manipulation, an external property. As Marcel notes, the observation that our possessions eat us up becomes false "when we are more vitally and actively bound up with something serving as the immediate subject-matter of a personal creative act, a subject-matter perpetually renewed . . . In all these cases, having tends, not to be destroyed, but to be sublimated and changed into being" (165). In releasing our possessive grasp, we have the possibility of seeing reality for what it is.

Each of these authors offers a way of finding meaning within the finite, the transient, and the temporal. They do not flinch from looking into the absurd or the abyss of death. Indeed, they take such a vision as a precondition for meaningful living. They center the significance of life precisely within its finitude and limits. One does not find meaning by escaping the limits of life but by full immersion into its most mundane details, accepting them and then mastering them and recognizing their finitude. On the other hand, through this process we also transcend these realities and encounter the possibility of discovering meaning in those events and experiences.

Religious Responses

Another response to meaning in the world in which we live is religious. To discuss this, I want to turn to some reflections developed from the theology of St. Bonaventure, the medieval Franciscan theologian. In doing so, I recognize that I am parting company with perhaps all of the transhumans, who typically reject religion. Nonetheless, I want to show how a vision that is accepting of the human condition, but not content with it, can provide other insights into life and offer a vision of hope. The section to follow shares an insight in common with the transhumanist movement—our hearts are restless—but agrees with Augustine, who says that they will be restless until they rest in God, rather than with the transhumanists, who think resting in nanoswarms will resolve our longings.

Bonaventure tells us that we have two books to read: the book of nature and the book of the scriptures. This suggests to me that the book of nature is insufficient in itself to give us the whole story, the complete text. There are gaps in the text that we need to fill in. In doing this we can reconstruct the whole text. There are a variety of other books of nature that we can and, I would suggest, must read, such as the books of anthropology, poetry, chemistry, and the other books that comprise the full library, each of which can complement our description and understanding of reality. Thus, Bonaventure affirms the value of nature and sees it as a complement to the other book we have been given. Here I want to focus on some added dimensions from the book on which Bonaventure focuses: the book of the scriptures.

Some consequences follow that are important to a consideration of the agenda of the transhumanist movement, particularly with regard to endless progress for the self and to living forever. First, we need to affirm that evolution is not the whole story. While evolution is a critical text, it clearly does not have a conclusion, or at least a conclusion that can be predicted from the opening chapters. In some ways it is the primordial never-ending story, a process that emerges and develops as it will. Yet the scriptures tell us we have a purpose, a goal, a consummation, in the phrase of Bonaventure. That goal is the completion of the circle begun in creation and fulfilled in the return of the world to the presence of the creator. While the how and when of this are unknown, the more critical aspect is the journey on which we currently find ourselves and how we conduct ourselves on that journey. For example, from an evolutionary perspective we can speak of genetic selfishness and competition of species. These are the inbuilt tendencies to seek the good of oneself and one's close relations so that one will gain a reproductive advantage. This seems to be demonstrated quite clearly by sociobiology and is part of the text of the book of nature. Yet when we turn to another book, the Christian scriptures, we have the injunction to love our enemies and to return good to those who would harm us. We are told to emphasize generosity, not competition. Here we have an example of how one text can add a story line to another text. The integration of these two story lines suggests the importance of two goods: the individual good and the common good. In our journey we need to attend to both, to avoid the dangers that come from, to use Bonaventure's phrase, being limited to one book only and being curved into oneself, his definition of the consequence of original sin. Clearly we need to attend to our good and the good of our families, but we also need to look beyond ourselves to the good of others around us. This perspective would suggest that in research we seek to benefit the common good and make the benefits of research available to those in need. This perspective would also influence research priorities, the kinds of research done—for example, public health issues versus genetic diseases influencing a small population—and perhaps how we price the products of research. It is clear that in the current dispensation, research follows money, and the money is generated from private corporations and venture capital as well as congressional allocations that in turn are substantively influenced by lobbying groups and celebrity spokespersons for various diseases. A perspective that highlights the common good may search for alternative ways to generate research priorities.

Readings from the scriptures as well as the Bonaventurian perspective of exemplarity give us additional general points of orientation as we continue to work our way through the complexities of genetic research. First is a rejection of philosophical reductionism. The elements of the natural world, as complex and exciting as they are, are not the whole picture. A religious, and particularly a Franciscan, perspective suggests that what we see is not the whole story. As fascinating as the book of nature is, there is another dimension to which that text alludes. The book of nature is a point of departure for the reader who, if he or she reads carefully, will discover a subtext or perhaps a hypertext buried within the book of nature. One such hypertext might be evolutionary surprise, the evolution of unforeseen or unpredicted species. Another might be sheer wonder at the reality of life itself, its power and its fecundity.

Second, the world of nature is not purely instrumental. While it is true that life lives on life and that various life forms come and go during the course of evolution's wanderings, nonetheless we humans have emerged from this process as editors of the text. As editors and readers of this book, we are horrified by those who burn books and prohibit publications in an attempt to suppress the truth they contain. How much more, then, should we respect the text of the book of nature. We must listen carefully to its multilayered messages, learn its interactions with other elements, and understand what new editions of this text will say to us as well as how our editing might indeed transform us as editors. Our text is a guide, and while slavish fidelity to the literal text will give mistaken readings, so too will an abandonment of the text.

Third, we need to focus on the common good as well as individual goods. In some ways we can understand the text of genetic selfishness as a model of this in that the individual is expected to sacrifice its life for the reproductive advantage of the kinship group. But this text needs to be complemented by the text of scripture, which tells us that our self-sacrifice needs to go far beyond the kinship group, beyond the strategy of tit for tat that can also be read from the book of nature. The scriptural injunction to love one's enemies is a radical reediting of some texts from the book of nature. The agenda is not reproductive advantage but the welfare of others, those with no relation to us—indeed, seeking the welfare of those who would harm us. Thus, an integrated reading of both books will help us establish the balance between the good of the group and the good of the larger community.

Conclusion

Reading the book of nature can help us in evaluating and establishing priorities. Thus, while health is important, is it the most important reality? Given that we know that life is finite, otherwise evolution would be at a rapid dead-end, and that we are on a journey elsewhere, where should we place our priorities in health care? Focused research to eliminate all disease? Basic research to expand our horizons? Public health needs? Child and elder care? Efforts to re-edit the text of the book of nature through genetic intervention offer many benefits: cure of disease, the availability of a supply of organs for human use, a larger and healthier food supply. Yet in our efforts to re-edit we must not totally instrumentalize or commodify the text or seek to privilege our species by attempting medical immortality. We know what happens when an author hits on a successful style or genre: the author and the editors seek to repeat it as often as possible and to an ever-larger audience. But we also know that sequels frequently fail to have the power of the original and that often the sequels are boring and even shoddy. This lesson from publishing might be a useful one as we think through the various genetic interventions being proposed. Will the intervention actually be beneficial, or will it simply be a pale and not too useful imitation of the original? Will the formula work for a few new texts but eventually show itself incapable of bearing a creative story line? Might this be a helpful analogy for thinking through the ethical issues associated with reproductive cloning? While reproductive cloning is understandable as a final attempt of artificial reproduction, some of the motives and intentions frequently associated with reproductive cloning could give rise to the problems associated with sequels. Cloning also by its nature freezes the status quo, provides a single page of the book of nature to be read over and over again. While the page will have meaning and worth because of the content in it, there is no development, no change, no inno-vation. When one comes to the end of a page, one instinctively turns it. With a clone, there is but one page.

Seeing the human as a reader from the Bonaventurian perspective does not resolve particular ethical problems in genetics. Yet this perspective reminds us that as readers we cannot read from one perspective only; we must be open to multiple, complementary, and multidisciplinary readings of this core text, the book of nature. To address our current problems we need to recognize the complexity of this text, its many layers of meanings, and also its deep openness to many levels of reality.

One ending can come from Bonaventure: "This is the whole of our meta-physics: it is about emanation, exemplarity, and consummation; that is, to be illumined by spiritual rays and to be led back to the Supreme Being."[2] While Bonaventure has in mind primarily a religious interpretation of this phrase, there is also a profoundly human meaning that can help us under-stand the significance of our moral lives. We are emanated in the sense that we emerge from our evolutionary past and bear the traces of that past in our very bodies. We are related to all creatures past and present. And our DNA, the living reality of that relation, is what will project us into the fu-ture. We are an exemplar in that who we are and how we live communi-cates a meaning of life to those around us. We have the opportunity to reveal the meaning of a good life, a life filled with wisdom, with concern for others, with affirming the dignity of the marginalized. Our lives can manifest a richness built out of our readings in the book of nature. And ultimately there will be a consummation. We will be returned to the primal elements out of which we originally came. Our DNA returns to reenter the great cycle of DNA. But in this there is renewal and transformation, the completion of our good journey. What we cannot forget, whether we ex-press this in religious language or not, is that the book of nature tells us that we have an origin, meaning, and significance. We are part of the text of nature, but we are also readers and speakers of this text. We are part of the alphabet on the basis of which new editions of the text can be based, but we are also in a profound relation to all such future editions. Thus, our status as humans is in profound solidarity with this book; our correspond-ing responsibility as readers is to give a clear and rich reading. And this reading will help us to generate a lifestyle—one totally contrary to the ad-ventures of transhumanism, but an adventure nonetheless.

Another ending is summed up directly and clearly by James Bacik (2005, 24) in a reflection on the significance of Karl Rahner's theology, a reflection, interestingly enough, that echoes some of the themes of Heidegger and Camus: "This Christian anthropology has 'the improbable optimism' to assert that average human beings who 'ply their way through life' can rise above the 'miserable narrow anxiety of their existence' and 'the banality of everyday life' by loving others through simple, unselfish acts of kindness, understanding, and compassion. By 'daring to risk' our own autonomy and freedom in genuine acts of love, we enter 'into the unfathomable, unbounded dwelling place of God.'"

Kurzweil in concert with the posthumanists and transhumanists notes that many improvements to us will be able to be downloaded through the Internet. "We won't even need a heart" (Linsay, 2005). And therein lies the entire problem of the transhumanist movement.

NOTES

1. For a further development of this idea, see Shannon, 2004.
2. See Bonaventure's *Sermons on the Six Days of Creation*, 3, 2 (V, 343).

REFERENCES

Alexander, B. 2003. *Rapture.* New York: Basic Books.
Bacik, J. 2005. Is Rahner obsolete? *Commonweal,* January 28.
Camus, A. 1955. The myth of Sisyphus. In *The Myth of Sisyphus and Other Essays.* New York: Random House.
Isherwoon, C. 2005. Sugarplum vision becomes a taunting specter. *New York Times,* February 25, B2.
Kurzweil, R. 2002. The evolution of mind in the twenty-first century. In *Are We Spiritual Machines?* ed. George Gilder and Jay Richards. Seattle: Discovery Institute Press.
Linsay, J. 2005. Inventor believes humans eventually will be immortal. *Seattle Times,* February 13. http://seattletimes.nwsource.com/html/nationworld/2002178868_immortal13.html.
Marcel, G. 1965. *Being and Having: An Existentialist Diary.* New York: Harper Torchbook.
More, M. 2003. Principles of extropy. Extropy Institute. www.extropy.com/principles.htm.

Shannon, T. A. 2004. How far should enhancement go? *Human Development* 25 (fall):36–43.

Vita-More, N. 1997. Workout schedule. www.natasha.cc/bodybuilder.htm.

Vita-More, N. 2005. Primo posthuman (2005 edition). www.natasha.cc/primo3m+ comparision.htm.

Yardley, J. 2005. Fearing future, China starts to give girls their due. *New York Times,* January 31, late edition, final, sec. A.

CHAPTER 5

Stem Cell Research and Intervention

ROBERT LANZA, M.D.

Stem cells raise the prospect of regenerating failing body parts and treating a wide range of disorders that result from tissue loss or dysfunction. More than 16 million patients worldwide have neurodegenerative disorders such as Parkinson and Alzheimer disease, more than 200 million people have diabetes, and millions more have cardiovascular disease, arthritis, AIDS, stroke, and other disorders that may one day be treatable using stem cell technology. In addition to generating functional replacement cells, there is the possibility that these cells could be used to reconstitute more complex tissues and organs, including blood vessels, bone, myocardial patches, and even entire organs, such as kidneys or hearts. In fact, it has been estimated that by 2010 more than 2 million people will have end-stage renal disease alone, at an aggregate cost of more than $1 trillion during the coming decade. Techniques such as somatic cell nuclear transfer (SCNT) could be used to eliminate the immune responses associated with the transplantation of these various tissues, and thus the requirement for immunosuppressive drugs or immunomodulatory protocols, which carry the risk of a wide variety of serious and potentially life-threatening complications.

Cloning Basics

Cloning is conceptually simple. In one technique, the nucleus (containing the DNA) of an egg cell is removed, and the somatic (body) cell to be cloned is placed under the zona pellucida (the thick envelope surrounding the egg) using a micropipette. An electrical charge is sent through the unit, which damages the membrane between the two cells so that the nucleus of the donor cell is dumped into the enucleated egg. The reconstructed egg cell is then fooled into thinking it has been fertilized by exposing it to certain chemicals. It starts to divide, and the result is an embryo ready to be implanted into a uterus. In animal *reproductive* cloning, this embryo can be implanted into a surrogate animal, where it can generate a live animal. Alternatively, the embryo can be put in a Petri dish to generate embryonic stem cells for cell therapy (*therapeutic* cloning).

Using this technology, we at Advanced Cell Technology (ACT) have cloned several animal species, including mice, cows, and even endangered species—and in 2001, we used this technology to generate the first (early stage) cloned human embryo (Cibelli et al., 2001). However, contrary to popular belief, cloning cells or an animal will not make a genetically identical copy of the donor. Cells have two genomes: the nuclear genome (the DNA contained in the chromosomes in the nucleus) and the mitochondrial genome (the DNA contained in the many mitochondria that reside in the cytoplasm). In the cloning procedure, the nuclear genome (the chromosomes) is removed from the egg cell, but the egg cell still contains the original mitochondrial genome. Numerous studies have shown that animals produced by cloning inherit their mitochondria entirely or in part from the recipient egg and not from the donor cell. (For the area of transplantation, this raises important questions about tissue rejection, as I will later discuss.)

Reversing Aging

For all the ability to created cloned animals and stem cells, one of the serious problems posed for transplant medicine is the age of the donor nucleus. Dolly, the first cloned sheep, died after a diagnosis of arthritis (Adam, 2002) and a report that she was prematurely old (Shiels et al., 1999). Such premature aging of transplanted cells would be a setback for the possibility of human therapeutic cloning: it would be unadvisable to take a cell from an elderly patient to generate new replacement cells that would be senescent (old and nondividing) and perhaps die within a few weeks or months once they were transplanted back into the patient. However, we published a paper in *Science* that showed that this is not the case, and that you can take an old decrepit cell and use SCNT to restore it to a phenotypically youthful state (Lanza et al., 2000b).

In our particular study, we set out to create cows that would produce human serum albumin (an important protein found in the blood) in their milk. We took cells from a 45-day-old fetus and introduced the necessary genetic construct to produce the human protein, grew up the cells, and then selected them with drugs. By the time the whole procedure was complete, we ended up with cells that were senescent or nearly senescent. If the Dolly myth was correct, these senescent cells would be useless, and you couldn't use them to generate a cloned animal. However, in our experiment a herd of animals were cloned from these senescent cells, animals that are now producing human serum albumin in their milk. Fetal growth and development require a substantial number of population doublings. Therefore, if you started with a senescent cell, you could not have ended up with these term animals if the age of the donor cell was reflected in the resulting clone.

Equally important is what we found when we looked inside the cells of these animals—in particular, at telomere length. Telomeres are the strands of DNA at the end of the chromosomes. They are like fuses that get shorter and shorter every time a cell divides, until eventually you reach a point where the cell can no longer divide. The telomere length of newborn calves is quite long, and as the animals grow older it gets shorter. The cloning procedure restored the telomeres not just to their normal length but to a length longer than their age-matched controls. So we know that, at least using our SCNT methodology, the cloning procedure can reverse the aging process and restore these cells to a state useful for medical therapy (Lanza et al., 2000b).

We also carried out other studies to verify that we didn't simply lengthen the telomeres without reversing cellular aging (Lanza et al., 2000b). For instance, we looked at the lifespan of the cloned cells. Fetal cells normally go through about 60 population doublings. In this study, we grew our cells to senescence—to the end of their lifespan. SCNT restored their lifespan to normal (in fact, to a greater lifespan). These results have important implications for transplant medicine.

The Medical Potential of Somatic Cell Nuclear Transfer

Neurodegenerative diseases cost the U.S. health care system more than $200 billion per year and are likely to be some of the first disorders treated using embryonic stem cell therapies. For instance, Parkinson disease affects half a million to a million people in the United States and a comparable number in Europe. The disease results in weakness, tremors, and disordered movements, which alternate with paralyzing immobility during the late stages. The symptoms are familiar: stooped posture; blank, unemotional, or "masked" face; stiffness and slowness of movement; small voice; and shuffled steps.

Parkinson disease affects the central nervous system, which is an immune-privileged site, so transplanting dopamine-producing cells (which we can generate from embryonic stem cells) would be much easier than, for example, trying to treat diabetes, which would involve dealing with the full immune system. Several years ago, we at ACT found that dopamine-producing neurons generated by nuclear transfer could be used to treat Parkinsonian symptoms in the rat (Zawada et al., 1998). When we transplanted cloned dopamine neurons back into the brains, the grafts were successful after two months. By looking at rotational behavior, the standard way scientists measure Parkinsonian symptoms in these animals, we found that the cloned cells reduced the clinical symptoms in half within 60 days. The hope is that we can achieve similar results in humans.

Another disease that could be treated with SCNT is type 1 diabetes. According to the World Health Organization, more than 200 million people worldwide have diabetes, and the incidence continues to increase by about 2 percent per year. Type 1 diabetes is due to an autoimmune destruction of the insulin-producing β-cells in the pancreas. This disease leads to increased risk of blindness, kidney failure, heart attack, stroke, and amputation due to advanced vascular disease. In the past, animal or recombinant human sources of insulin have provided the replacement therapy required by persons with type 1 diabetes. Unfortunately, injected insulin cannot precisely mimic the ability of the normal pancreas to regulate blood glucose concentrations. The concentration of insulin in the blood is normally linked to the blood glucose concentrations by moment-to-moment fluctuations in insulin secretion by the β-cells. These fluctuations, which serve to control blood glucose concentrations, depend on a complex series of biochemical pathways in the living β-cells and are currently difficult or impossible to simulate by insulin injection. The results of the Diabetes Control and Complications Trial (DCCT) suggest that failure to achieve physiologic glucose control with injected insulin is responsible for the serious complications of this disease.

There is hope that the transplantation of β-cells will not only eliminate the need for daily insulin injections but also prove effective in preventing or retarding the development of the complications associated with diabetes. One possible approach is to transplant the entire pancreas, but in the United States only a few thousand usable pancreases are available, and millions of people with diabetes could benefit from the therapy. Whole pancreas transplantation also requires major vascular surgery as well as a lifetime of immunosuppression, which carries the risk of serious and potentially life-threatening complications.

An alternative to whole organ transplantation is to transplant just pancreatic islets. The pancreas is mainly a digestive organ, and only 1 or 2 percent of the cells are the so-called islets of Langerhans, which contain the β-cells that produce insulin. The islets can be isolated from the pancreas using enzymatic or mechanical digestion procedures, and then injected back into the liver or spleen to treat diabetes. But isolating islets only exacerbates the problem of organ supply: two to eight glands are necessary to obtain a sufficient β-cell mass to reverse diabetes. Also, this approach is like the razorblade business: because islets have a finite lifespan, it is necessary to retransplant every few months or years. This approach, then, is not overly practical, not only because of the serious shortage of donor organs but also because islet transplantation—like whole organ transplantation—requires generalized immunosuppression.

A number of other strategies have been tried. For example, we've used microcapsules to separate the transplanted islet tissue from the immune system of the body using synthetic, selectively permeable barriers. We've succeeded in reversing diabetes in mice, rats, rabbits, and even dogs using this approach, but it doesn't solve the problem of organ shortage. In addition, the capsules must be implanted in the peritoneum or other body sites, which poses considerable difficulties in both the long and short terms, including risk of peritonitis, organ scarring, adhesions, and infection.

SCNT could potentially solve these problems. When I first began cell transplant research, we were just learning how to isolate the human islets from the pancreas. A pancreas that had been removed from a patient with pancreatitis was examined in the laboratory. The gland was very fibrotic, and we were able to isolate only about 50,000 to 100,000 islets, while a normal human pancreas contains half a million to a million islets. When we injected the islets back into the patient's portal vein, he was cured of diabetes. That procedure (transplanting one's own cells back into oneself) is known as an autograft. It has now been done dozens and dozens of times, and it works most of the time. Those results stand in sharp contrast to the worldwide experience using islet allotransplants (i.e., islets transplanted from one patient into another). Before the recent Edmonton Protocol, only approximately 8 percent of such patients achieved insulin independence— and often only for a few weeks or months—despite transplanting more than a million islets in many cases.

So what's the difference between these two scenarios? Why did a handful of islets from the patient with pancreatitis reverse diabetes, whereas the majority of allogenic transplants fail? The answer, of course, is that the patient with pancreatitis got his own cells back. And that's exactly what SCNT aims to do. One takes a cell from the patient and fuses it with an enucleated egg to generate embryonic stem (ES) cells. Those cells can then be coaxed into various replacement cell types in the laboratory, such as neurons, cardiomyocytes, or islets.

Generating Stem Cells, Tissues, and Organs for Therapy

We published a paper in *Science* that demonstrated how the nuclear transfer (cloning) procedure can be skipped by using "parthenogenetic activation" (Cibelli et al., 2002). An egg cell is "fooled" into thinking it is fertilized; after a few cleavage divisions, a blastocystlike "parthenote" is obtained, from which embryonic stem cells can be generated. These parthenogenetic stem cells can then be turned into the various replacement cells. We have generated stem cells from a monkey that are capable of turning into cells from all three germ layers. By modifying their environment, we've been able to turn them into neurons, gut, hair follicles, bone, and even hematopoietic (blood cell) precursors. For instance, we generated beating heart cells in one dish and contracting smooth muscle in another. Yet another plate was almost thrown away because it looked as if it were contaminated with bacteria undergoing Brownian movement. When placed under the microscope, it turned out to contain hundreds of beating ciliated epithelial cells. These stem cells seem to do all sorts of incredible things effortlessly. In fact, we can generate entire dishes full of dopaminergic neurons that could potentially be used to treat Parkinson disease. We're just starting to learn some of the tricks needed to get the cells to do what we want. For example, mouse embryonic stem cells have been turned into a pure population of heart cells. When the cells were injected back into the heart of a mouse, they were found to have formed stable intracardiac grafts.

In addition to using SCNT to generate replacement cells and tissues in the laboratory, we've carried out a number of exciting experiments in animals. For instance, we scoured the country to locate old cows (equivalent to humans around 70 years old) and used nuclear transfer to give them new immune cells. We took skin cells from their ears and, using nuclear transplantation, generated new youthful immune cells that were infused back into the animals (Lanza et al., 2005). However, our goal wasn't simply to give an old cow a new immune system. In humans there are more than 80 autoimmune disorders, such as multiple sclerosis, rheumatoid arthritis, and lupus. If we can get this technology to work, we may be able to reboot a patient's immune system and give him or her back new immune cells minus whatever environmental insult may have caused the disorder. The potential could be enormous, not only as a cure for various autoimmune diseases. The same cells that give rise to the immune system also give rise to hematopoietic stem cells. We know from rodent and human studies that these cells can be used to treat arthritis. If they are infused into an infarcted heart or into the bloodstream of an animal after a heart attack, they can create new myocardium and vasculature. In fact, it may also be possible to inject these youthful precursor cells into an elderly person to prevent pneumonia or cancer, without any need for drugs.

The body of scientific literature suggests that hematopoietic stem cells play a general reparative role in the body. A paper in the *New England Journal of Medicine* showed that up to 7 percent of the cells in female hearts transplanted into men had a Y chromosome. Presumably, the hematopoietic stem cells circulating in the male patient's body maintained and repaired the hearts (Quaini et al., 2002). Our *Science* paper indicated that the cloning procedure resets the clock of cells by elongating their telomeres (Lanza et al., 2000b). Therefore, if you injected cloned precursor cells into an adult, you should have a competitive population of cells (much like fetal/neonatal hematopoietic stem cells) that would circulate throughout the body and repair damaged areas of the heart or repair damage from a stroke or arthritis. It sounds like a magic elixir, but it may well be real. The rodent studies look promising.

But for all of the promise of individual or small groups of cells, to realize the full potential of therapeutic cloning it will be important to understand how to reconstitute the cells into more complex tissues and structures. Although SCNT could eliminate the problem of immune incompatibility, the task of putting the cells together to create or recreate functional structures—an area know as tissue engineering—remains. The basic concept of tissue engineering is to use biodegradable materials and/or self-assembly principles to regenerate more complex structures. For relatively simple tissues, such as skin and blood vessel substitutes, this may involve seeding cells onto masses or sheets of polymeric scaffold. There are machines that allow us to create scaffolds of any shape and design.

Creating vital organs, such as the kidney, the liver, or even the heart, however, will be a much greater scientific challenge and will require assembling different cell types and materials with great combinatorial and architectural complexity. The first organ that was tissue engineered was a bladder that was grown in the laboratory of Anthony Atala at Harvard University and Children's Hospital in Boston. These bladders were transplanted back into dogs and actually worked. In fact, we have a number of collaborations ongoing with Dr. Atala's group, and we published a paper in *Nature Biotechnology* that furnishes the first scientific evidence that SCNT actually works in the large-animal model with a sophisticated immune system similar to humans (Lanza et al., 2002). An important concern about using therapeutic cloning is the maternal mitochondrial DNA, alluded to above. Animals produced by cloning do not inherit their mitochondrial DNA from the clone donor, which raises questions of whether nonself mitochondrial proteins (synthesized by the mitochondrial DNA) in the cloned cells could stimulate an immune response after transplantation, thus defeating the main objective of the procedure. In rodents we know that this DNA can result in a loss of histocompatibility.

Therefore, there were questions of whether SCNT would really work or not. We carried out a study to see whether or not this immune response actually occurs. Using cloning, we created cardiac "patches," which could be used to fix the heart, and generated miniature kidneys. The ability to generate immunologically compatible cells using SCNT would overcome one of the major scientific challenges in transplantation medicine—namely, the problem of organ and tissue rejection.

We found that the cloned tissues all survived despite the presence of the foreign DNA. In the kidney study, not only did the renal units survive and function as kidneys, but also immunological studies carried out both in the transplanted animals and in the laboratory confirmed that there was no rejection response to the cloned tissues. The results were impressive: the kidneys produced straw-yellow urine. In fact, the kidneys removed toxic waste products from the blood (such as urea, nitrogen, and creatinine) at a level up to 60 percent of what is considered normal in urine. The heart patches showed well-organized cellular structures, whereas the non-cloned patches had been reduced to debris as a result of rejection. We also carried out a delayed-type hypersensitivity (DTH) test, which is considered the best test for detecting an immunological response to transplanted tissue (short of outright transplant rejection). There was a clear immune response to the control allogenic cells (i.e., to cells that were transplanted from genetically unrelated animals). However, we were unable to detect any immune response against the cloned tissue. These results were corroborated using various laboratory tests, such as the Elispot assay, which estimated the response of the animal's blood cells to stimulation by the cloned and control cells. Again, the results confirmed that there was no rejection response to the cloned cells.

Conclusion

Two major problems exist in transplantation medicine: immune rejection and organ shortage. Our results suggest that it may be possible to overcome both of these hurdles with stem cell technology. In addition to generating immune-compatible tissues, it is possible to bioengineer cloned cells into complex functional structures such as heart patches and kidneys. A staged, developmental strategy will be required to achieve this ultimate goal. The kidney performs some of the most critical functions necessary for survival, and it is likely to require substantial additional effort to generate a tissue-engineered kidney that can actually be transplanted into a patient.

But for all the medical promise of cloning technology, there is considerable controversy. SCNT requires the creation and disaggregation of pre-implantation-stage embryos to generate embryonic stem cells (Lanza et al., 2000a). Although the embryo does not have human form or sentience at this stage—in fact, there isn't a single somatic or body cell present yet—some believe that human "personhood," and thus claims of moral status and dignity, begins at fertilization, or, in the case of cloning, at the genetic beginning. To subvert the development of a potential human being would be considered morally objectionable. To others, the primitive streak is the first trace of the embryo. This does not occur until the end of the second week after fertilization when implantation is under way. Before this stage, twinning and recombination are possible, and developmental individuality or "personhood" has not been established.

The potential therapeutic benefits of the procedure, it has been argued, far outweigh the harm. Where is the morality in letting millions of people continue to suffer from chronic and life-threatening disease? Yes, a human "pre-embryo" should be treated with respect. But does a completely undifferentiated ball of cells, one that is smaller than the head of pin, warrant the same rights and reverence as that accorded a living soul—a parent, a child or a partner—who might die because we fail to use this technology? This is not just an academic ethical question; a real human tragedy is out there. One day, millions of patients could benefit from this technology.

REFERENCES

Adam, D. 2002. Clone pioneer calls for health tests. *Nature* 415:103.
Cibelli, J., et al. 2001. Somatic cell nuclear transfer in humans: Pronuclear and early embryonic development *Journal of Regenerative Medicine* 2:25.
Cibelli, J. B., K. A. Grant, K. B. Chapman, K. Cuniff, T. Worst, H. L. Green, S. J. Walker, et al. 2002. Parthenogenetic stem cells in nonhuman primates. *Science* 295:819.
Lanza, R. P., A. L. Caplan, L. M. Silver, J. B. Cibelli, M. D. West, and R. M. Green. 2000a. The ethical validity of using nuclear transfer in human transplantation. *Journal of the American Medical Association* 284:3175–79.
Lanza, R. P., J. B Cibelli, C. Blackwell, V. J. Cristofalo, M. K. Francis, G. M. Baerlocher, et al. 2000b. Extension of cell life-span and telomere length in animals cloned from senescent somatic cells. *Science* 288:665–69.

Lanza, R. P., H. Y. Chung, J. J. Yoo, P. J. Wettstein, C. Blackwell, N. Borson, E. Hofmeister, et al. 2002. Generation of histocompatible tissues using nuclear transplantation. *Nature Biotechnology* 20;689–96

Lanza, R. P., J. H. Shieh, P. J. Wettstein, R. W. Sweeney, K. Wu, A. Weisz, N. Borson, et al. 2005. Long-term bovine hematopoietic engraftment with clone-derived stem cells. *Cloning and Stem Cells* 7:95–106.

Quaini, F., K. Urbanek, A. P. Beltrami, N. Finato, C. A. Beltrami, B. Nadal-Ginard, J. Kajstura, et al. 2002. Chimerism of the transplanted heart. *New England Journal of Medicine* 346:5–15.

Shiels, P., A. J. Kind, K. H. Campbell, D. Waddington, I. Wilmut, A. Colman, and A. E. Schnieke. 1999. Analysis of telomere lengths in cloned sheep. *Nature* 399: 316–17.

Zawada, W., J. B. Michael, P. K. Cibelli, E. D. Choi, P. J. Clarkson, S. E. Golueke, et al. 1998. Cloned transgenic bovine neurons for transplantation in Parkinsonian rats. *Nature Medicine* 4:569–74.

CHAPTER 6

The Ethical, Legal, and Social Implications of Antiaging Technologies

MAXWELL J. MEHLMAN, J.D.

This chapter addresses three main issues that continue the discussion of technology in an aging society. First, what should be the goal of antiaging technologies? Second, should they be thought of as therapies or enhancements, and what difference does it make? Third, how should these technologies be regulated?

What Should Be the Goal of Antiaging Technologies?

There are three possible goals of antiaging technologies. One is "compressed morbidity" (Fries, 1980). The idea is to lead long lives free of chronic disease and disability, and then die rather quickly as people reach the natural limits of the human lifespan. Arguably this represents the main goal of geriatric medicine and of many gerontologists, who strive to combat the ravages of disease in their older patients.

A second potential antiaging objective is "decelerated aging" (Olshansky, Hayflick, and Carnes, 2002). This can take the form of prolonged youthfulness or vigor, or it can combine youthful vigor with an extension of the lifespan. The ultimate realization would be "arrested aging": eternal, or at least extremely prolonged, youth, the long-sought brass ring of antiaging enthusiasts. Ever since the medieval alchemists began searching for a "philosopher's stone" to confer immortality, there has been an energetic discussion of the pros and cons of decelerated aging, but in practice few people are likely to reject the prospect of a prolonged youthful lifespan.

But there is a third possible outcome of antiaging efforts: simply prolonging the human lifespan. There has been considerable interest in this objective among antiaging researchers, if only as a scientific accomplishment. For instance, there has been a vigorous effort to confound Leonard Hayflick's (2001) prediction that cells are programmed to divide no more than 50 times (the so-called Hayflick limit), which would impose a genetic limit on the lifespan of any organism. However, as many commentators have recognized, extending lifespan is hardly desirable if it merely allows the individual to suffer the illnesses and debilities of old age for a longer period. In a previous article, my colleagues and I referred to this as a state of "prolonged senescence" (Juengst et al., 2003). Natural aging advocate Francis Fukuyama (2002) calls it the "national nursing home scenario," in which people routinely live to be 150 but spend the last 50 years in a state of childlike dependence on caretakers. And who can forget Jonathan Swift's parody of prolonged senescence in his account of the Struldbrugs in *Gulliver's Travels:*

> When they came to fourscore years, which is reckoned the extremity of living in this country, they had not only all the follies and infirmities of other old men, but many more which arose from the dreadful prospect of never dying. They were not only opinionative, peevish, covetous, morose, vain, talkative, but incapable of friendship, and dead to all natural affection, which never descended below their grandchildren. Envy and impotent desires are their prevailing passions. But those objects against which their envy seems principally directed, are the vices of the younger sort and the deaths of the old. By reflecting on the former, they find themselves cut off from all possibility of pleasure; and whenever they see a funeral, they lament and repine that others have gone to a harbour of rest to which they themselves never can hope to arrive. They have no remembrance of anything but what they learned and observed in their youth and middle-age, and even that is very imperfect; and for the truth or particulars of any fact, it is safer to depend on common tradition, than upon their best recollections . . . At ninety, they lose their

teeth and hair; they have at that age no distinction of taste, but eat and drink whatever they can get, without relish or appetite. The diseases they were subject to still continue, without increasing or diminishing. In talking, they forget the common appellation of things, and the names of persons, even of those who are their nearest friends and relations. For the same reason, they never can amuse themselves with reading, because their memory will not serve to carry them from the beginning of a sentence to the end; and by this defect, they are deprived of the only entertainment whereof they might otherwise be capable. (Swift, 1796)

While it might seem silly for anyone to embrace the prospect of such a dismal future, the spectacle surrounding the death of Terri Schiavo illustrates the temptation to value living longer regardless of the quality of life. Not only must individuals have the right to end their lives when the right time comes, but also funding entities and researchers must avoid pursuing projects that aim to prolong life merely for life's sake.

Antiaging Technologies: Therapies or Enhancements?

The next major question concerning antiaging efforts is whether they should be regarded as therapies or enhancements. This is not merely a theoretical excursion for philosophers of science. The answer has important practical consequences. In the first place, neither public nor private health insurance in the United States pays for biomedical enhancement. This policy originated in response to cosmetic surgery, and while it can be circumvented to some extent by physicians willing to submit fraudulent bills for enhancement while calling it therapy, insurers constantly strive to detect and thwart this practice. In short, if antiaging interventions are regarded as enhancements, then most people who obtain them will have to pay for them out of pocket. Depending on how expensive they are, this could mean that life extension will be available only to the relatively well off.

There is also a third way to conceive of antiaging interventions: as preventive measures. If aging is deemed a pathological process, then regarding antiaging interventions as "preventive" confers on them a preferred policy status, because prevention generally is considered superior to treatment. On the other hand, preventive health-related measures traditionally have been the purview of the public health system. This system is marked by less deference to patient and physician decision-making autonomy than ordinary medical care. Public health authorities routinely override privacy and confidentiality in order to control transmissible diseases, and they are vested with the ability to confine and forcibly treat individuals without the due process that ordinarily accompanies government coercion. The upshot is that if public officials gather preventive antiaging technologies under a public health umbrella, these technologies could be subject to much greater public control than if they were regarded as enhancements.

Another problem that arises if antiaging interventions are regarded as enhancements is that they may be illegal. Fueled by the hysterical reaction to the use of steroids by athletes, we are in the midst of a war on biomedical enhancement that threatens to become as draconian as its parent War on Drugs. For example, Congress in 1988 made it a felony to distribute or possess with the intent to distribute human growth hormone "for any use in humans other than the treatment of disease or other recognized medical condition" (21 U.S.C. §333[e][1]). The U.S. Food and Drug Administration has already taken regulatory action under this law against companies hawking what the companies claim is human growth hormone for antiaging purposes (U.S. Food and Drug Administration, 2004). If combating aging is considered enhancement, then those who take human growth hormone for this purpose are committing a crime. As the war on enhancement expands, other antiaging interventions may fall under the same type of prohibition.

The key to whether antiaging interventions are considered enhancements or therapies is how the aging process itself is characterized. On the one hand, biogerontologists are adamant that aging is a natural rather than a pathological biological process. Leonard Hayflick argues, for example, that "aging is not a disease, so the concept of seeking a cure for it is tantamount to seeking a cure for embryogenesis or child or adult development" (Hayflick, 2001, 20). On the other hand, even biogerontologists like Hayflick acknowledge that aging is the greatest risk factor for the leading causes of death and morbidity (Olshansky, Hayflick, and Carnes, 2002), and it is often difficult to separate the aging process itself from the deterioration that it causes. If aging is a disease, a pathological process, or even just a state that makes people susceptible to morbidities, then efforts to combat it can be deemed therapy. But if aging is a natural, even a desirable process, as people like Leon Kass, former chairman of the President's Council on

Bioethics, and Daniel Callahan, former president of the Hastings Center, believe, then efforts to interrupt its course are, at best, enhancements.[1]

How Should Antiaging Technologies Be Regulated?

The final issue is how to regulate antiaging technologies. Currently marketed antiaging products raise a number of regulatory concerns. They may be unsafe, causing harm to their users. They may be ineffective. Ineffective antiaging interventions that did not produce direct harm to users would still create a safety problem if they were used in place of effective interventions, for example, in lieu of effective treatments to treat age-associated pathologies. Ineffective antiaging interventions also defraud consumers, a concern especially with poor and elderly persons, who may be particularly vulnerable to unsupported marketing claims and who may lack adequate resources for basic necessities.

At the federal level, the Food and Drug Administration bears the responsibility for assuring the safety and efficacy of medical products. Antiaging interventions present the agency with difficult regulatory challenges. Some antiaging interventions, like caloric restriction, arguably lie outside the FDA's current legal authority because they constitute the practice of medicine rather than involving the use of a drug or medical device (Kessler, 1989). The practice of medicine is subject to regulation by the states, but there are numerous gaps and weaknesses in the system of state oversight, and a report by the General Accounting Office found that "in general [the states] focused little attention on antiaging and alternative medicine products" (U.S. General Accounting Office, 2001).

Another impediment to effective FDA regulation of antiaging interventions is the Dietary Supplement Health and Education Act (DSHEA), enacted in 1994, which allows certain antiaging interventions to be marketed as "dietary supplements" without proof of safety or efficacy. The definition of a dietary supplement in the act is extremely broad; virtually any antiaging substance qualifies so long as it does not make claims to treat a specific disease, bears a disclaimer on the label that the product is not approved by the FDA, and is taken by mouth (Federal Food, Drug, and Cosmetic Act, 21 U.S.C. §321[ff][1]). Before DSHEA, a product that claimed, for example, to "provide you with increased energy level, increased sex drive, improved skin texture, increased muscle mass, decreased body fat, decreased cholesterol, improved cognitive thinking skills, improved immune system, improved sleep patterns, and improved bone density" (Hormonal Antiaging Center, 2002) would have been regulated as a drug because it claims to affect the structure or function of the body (Federal Food, Drug, and Cosmetic Act, 21 U.S.C. §321[g][1][C]). But these claims can now be made for dietary supplements under DSHEA. Moreover, the dietary supplement laws reverse the traditional process for proving safety and efficacy. While the manufacturer of a new drug or medical device is required to establish safety and efficacy before marketing, the burden has been shifted to the FDA to show that a dietary supplement is unsafe before it can take action to restrict its sale or remove it from the market. Finally, unlike manufacturers of drugs and medical devices, manufacturers of dietary supplements are not required to disclose information about adverse events to the FDA, and little voluntary reporting takes place (U.S. General Accounting Office, 2001).

Even antiaging interventions that are clearly prescription drugs or medical devices may be able to escape FDA oversight when employed for unapproved antiaging purposes, because the Federal Food, Drug, and Cosmetic Act does not restrict physician prescribing of products for "off-label" uses. (However, the manufacturer of a drug or device must notify the FDA of adverse event reports stemming from off-label use [U.S. Department of Health and Human Services, 2001]). Historically, the agency has attempted to prohibit manufacturers from promoting their products for off-label uses, but since the passage of the FDA Modernization Act of 1997, manufacturers may distribute promotional materials for unapproved uses so long as they are in the process of seeking approval. In addition, the earlier FDA restrictions have been challenged in court as a violation of the manufacturer's First Amendment right to freedom of commercial speech (*Washington Legal Foundation v. Friedman,* 1998).

Another factor complicating the regulation of antiaging interventions is the controversy mentioned earlier over whether aging is a disease or a natural process. If aging is regarded as a natural process, then antiaging interventions are not therapies but enhancements, similar to cosmetic medicine. One consequence from a regulatory standpoint is that products that made antiaging claims could be marketed as dietary supplements because they would not be making claims to treat a specific disease. If they did not qualify as dietary supplements—for example, because they were not orally ingested—they would be drugs or medical devices, and regardless of whether they were regarded as therapies or as enhancements, they would have to have proof of safety and efficacy before they could be marketed. But the FDA's experience with cosmetic medicine, including nonprescription contact lenses, breast implants, liposuction, and Botox, demonstrates the difficulty outside of the therapeutic context of measuring efficacy and of comparing risks and benefits (Mehlman, 1999). The therapeutic/enhancement distinction is important for another reason as well: if antiaging interventions were regarded as enhancements, health insurers would not cover them, and this would remove the manufacturers' incentive to generate safety and efficacy data in order to convince insurers that their products should be covered because they are no longer experimental.

Efforts to protect consumer from unsafe antiaging interventions are also limited by the ease with which manufacturers and distributors can reach potential customers via electronic media. Television commercials and infomercials for antiaging interventions abound. Casual surfing of the Internet reveals innumerable websites hawking antiaging products and services. The Federal Trade Commission reviews advertising claims to make sure they are truthful and to prevent consumer injury, but it can do only so much. Its most notable effort to police questionable claims on the Internet is "Operation Cure-All," which consisted of two Internet surfs in 1997–98 that netted more than 1,600 sites worldwide and 800 sites in the United States alone, but the agency itself admits that this was only "the tip of the iceberg" (Beales, 2001).

Government regulatory efforts are supplemented by private action. Professional societies can issue policy statements about the dangers of misuse and take action against members who violate the organization's codes of ethics. Private individuals can sue physicians who prescribe unproven antiaging interventions that cause injury. But confirmed believers in antiaging interventions will not heed mainstream professional organizations, and malpractice suits are an inefficient and embattled technique for preventing patient harm.

While the major concern about antiaging interventions is that they may be detrimental to health, even relatively innocuous antiaging interventions can cause economic injury if consumers purchase them in the mistaken belief that they have been shown to be effective. There are no reliable estimates of how much money people spend on antiaging interventions, but the U.S. General Accounting Office believes that it is substantial (U.S. General Accounting Office, 2001). Consumers are vulnerable to two types

of quackery. One is straightforward fraud: selling products that the purveyors know to be ineffective. The challenge for government regulators is
to identify the perpetrators and apprehend them, their products, and their
assets. The other type of economic injury is caused by individuals who
market products in the true belief that they work, even though scientific
evidence is contradictory or lacking. Protecting consumers from this type
of economic injury is more difficult than preventing outright fraud. It may
be difficult to distinguish between a biological and a placebo effect. Moreover, the practice of medicine must remain open to new approaches. Physicians must be able to deviate from the mainstream without necessarily
violating the law or being liable for malpractice. The challenge is to distinguish between legitimate trial-and-error and quackery. Tell-tale signs of
the latter are physicians who earn substantial sums of money by selling
unproven products or services and do not participate in clinical trials.
Unfortunately, this appears to characterize a substantial segment of the
market.

Ultimately, marketers of antiaging interventions flourish because of a
basic tension in American social thought between paternalistic consumer
protection on the one hand and individual liberty and freedom of choice
on the other. Advocates of free choice—including the choice to employ
antiaging interventions—assert that individuals must be allowed to make
their own decisions about what to do with their own bodies, including
taking risks both known and unknown. Antiaging interventions also are
riding the crest of the wave of popular interest in alternative and complementary medicine generally. Growing numbers of consumers are turning
to these modalities in frustration at the slow progress of traditional medicine in combating many major diseases. Physicians and other health care
professionals find them a lucrative source of supplementary income, which
is especially welcome in an era of managed care. Even strident marketing
efforts for antiaging interventions may not offend consumers, because mainstream health care medicine increasingly appears to patients to be a commercial rather than a caring enterprise.

In conclusion, the question is how society should regulate antiaging
interventions to minimize the potential harm to consumers and to society
in general. Currently, the antiaging industry is able to flourish in a virtual
laissez-faire regulatory environment, with little obligation to provide safety
and efficacy information. This is likely to persist if antiaging technologies

are viewed as enhancements rather than as treatments or prevention. But even increased evidence of safety and efficacy will not alleviate social and ethical concerns. The more effective the intervention, the less the concern with hucksterism, but the greater the problem of unequal access and the prospect that individuals will subject themselves to unreasonable health risks in return for a chance to receive the perceived benefits of the technology. Not only would this cause harm to the individual; it would also impose costs on society that may not be outweighed by the societal benefits from living longer and healthier lives.

NOTE

1. Kass states that "to covet a prolonged life span for ourselves is both a sign and a cause of our failure to open ourselves to . . . any higher . . . purpose" (Kass, 1985, 316). Callahan states that "death is an inherent part of all life and is necessary for the continuation and vitality of species" (Callahan, 2000, 654).

REFERENCES

Beales, H. 2001. Testimony of the Federal Trade Commission before the U.S. Senate Special Committee on Aging, Washington, DC. www.ftc.gov/os/2001/09/healthfraud.htm.

Callahan, D. 2000. Death and the research imperative. *New England Journal of Medicine* 342:654–56.

Fries, J. F. 1980. Aging, natural death, and the compression of morbidity. *New England Journal of Medicine* 303:130–35.

Fukuyama, F. 2002. *Our Posthuman Future.* New York: Picador.

Hayflick, L. 2001. Anti-aging medicine: Hype, hope, and reality. *Generations* 25(4): 20–26.

Hormonal Antiaging Center. 2002. www.hormonalantiagingcenter.com/.

Juengst, E. T., R. H. Binstock, M. Mehlman, S. G. Post, and P. J. Whitehouse. 2003. Biogerontology, "anti-aging medicine," and the challenges of human enhancement. *Hastings Center Report,* July–August, 21–30.

Kass, L. 1985. *Toward a More Natural Science: Biology and Human Affairs.* New York: Free Press.

Kessler, D. A. 1989. The regulation of investigational drugs. *New England Journal of Medicine* 320:281.

Mehlman, M. J. 1999. Regulating genetic enhancement. *Wake Forest Law Review* 34:671–714.

Olshansky, J. S., L. Hayflick, and B. A. Carnes. 2002. Position statement on human aging. *Journals of Gerontology Series A: Biological Sciences and Medical Sciences* 57:B292–97.

Swift, J. 1726. *Gulliver's Travels,* ed. Henry Morely. London: George Routledge and Sons, 1906.

U.S. Department of Health and Human Services. 2001. Guidance for industry: Postmarketing safety reporting for human drug and biological products including vaccines.

U.S. Food and Drug Administration. 2004. Warning letter to Global Internet Alliance, February 18. www.fda.gov/foi/warning_letters/g4543d.htm.

U.S. General Accounting Office. 2001. Health products for seniors: Anti-aging products pose potential for physical and economic harm. GAO 01-1129.

Washington Legal Foundation v. Friedman, 13 F. Supp.2d 51 (D.D.C. 1998).

CHAPTER 7

Stem Cells and Aging

Quality and Quantity of Life in an Unjust World

KAREN LEBACQZ, PH.D.

Stem cell research offers two important and ethically very different possibilities for an aging society: (1) better quality of life in old age and (2) prolonged or extended life. Technologies that improve the quality of life in old age are not generally problematic, but those technologies that also extend or prolong life raise difficult ethical issues pertaining to justice.

Ethics and Quality of Life

Some stem cell therapies will have little effect on the length of life and can rather be expected to improve the quality of life. Before his death, my father had macular degeneration. As he lived alone following my mother's death, loss of his eyesight was a tremendous burden: he could no longer drive to doctors' appointments or to the grocery store, he could not see to pay his bills or file his paperwork, he could not read a newspaper or watch television. A stubborn and independent man, he felt keenly the loss of his eyesight and the accompanying loss of independence.

I have some appreciation of what he must have experienced. Several years ago, I went blind for a short duration. While my situation was *neu-rologically* different from macular degeneration, I suspect that what I *experienced* was similar to the experience of macular degeneration. (However, it happened over the course of a few days rather than a few years.) It began with an inability to see my own face in the mirror. Putting on makeup became a guessing game. I could not read, could not watch television, and could not drive. Worse yet, my old cat needed daily fluid injections, and I could not see the marks on the bottle to be sure that I was giving her the correct amount of fluid. Like my father, I am rather stubborn and independent. The loss of eyesight tested my ability to live alone and tested my faith and my sense of identity, particularly because I am a photographer in my spare time. Undergoing that experience has given me true empathy for the plight of older people with macular degeneration as well as some fears of what lies ahead in my own future.

Macular degeneration is a condition for which stem cell technologies offer significant hope of improvement or restoration of quality of life. Stem cell therapies might have enabled my father to keep his eyesight, to continue driving, to preserve his independence and his sense of dignity. Restoring the macula would not have extended his life (he died from cardiac failure), but it would have significantly improved what he perceived as the quality of his life. I sincerely hope that by the time I experience macular degeneration, stem cell technologies will offer a way to reverse such deterioration.

Therapies that improve the quality of life in this way without extending the lifespan seem to me to raise few new ethical issues. Stem cell research in general has already raised some ethical questions that have been debated at length in the literature (Holland, Lebacqz, and Zoloth, 2001; Snow, 2003). These questions include: (1) Is it ethical to do human embryonic[1] stem cell research at all, given the fact that such research destroys embryos? (2) What does justice require with regard to the availability and distribution of stem cell therapies? (3) Should public funds be used to support this research?[2] Any use of stem cell technology to derive new therapies must grapple with these fundamental questions, but they are not unique to the field of aging and stem cell technologies.

Of these general questions, the one that may have some particular applicability to the use of stem cells to improve quality of life in aging is the question about justice. As much as I would want a therapy for macular degeneration, I know that it would not be fair for me to have access to such therapy when others do not have access simply because I am better off financially than others are.[3] If the injustices that currently permeate our health care system are perpetuated, then stem cell therapies are also likely to be distributed in unjust ways. For me, this is a serious ethical issue. But it is not an issue unique to stem cell technologies, or to issues of aging. Therefore, it is important to ask whether there are some types of stem cell therapies that *do* raise particular questions related to aging.

Ethics and Quantity of Life

I think there are. Some stem cell therapies will not simply improve the *quality* of life for an aging society but are likely also to extend the *quantity* or *span* of life, enabling people to live not just *better* but *longer*. Using heart disease as an example, Lanza and Rosenthal (2004) note that there is promising research in animals: partially differentiated stem cells from a cloned mouse embryo were injected into the donor mouse's heart, "where they homed in on the site of injury from a heart attack, replacing 38 percent of the scar with healthy heart tissue within a month" (94). Should similar or better results occur in humans, it is likely that stem cells repairing heart tissue will not only improve the quality of life (e.g., by restoring mobility or ease of breathing) but also prevent many deaths and prolong many lives. In a German study of patients with severe heart damage following myocardial infarction, the patient's own heart progenitor cells were infused into the damaged artery; within four months the size of the damaged swath had diminished by more than one-third, and the patient's heart function had increased by 10 percent (Lanza and Rosenthal, 2004). While these results are preliminary and there are many technical as well as ethical issues to be worked out in stem cell research, the implications of these studies are exciting. Heart disease is the primary medical killer of women in the United States. From a feminist perspective of concern for women's lives and well-being,[4] stem cell research offers exciting possibilities for improving and even for saving women's lives.

Yet from an ethical perspective, it seems clear that interventions that offer not only improvement in *quality* of life but also the likelihood of extended *quantity* of life raise different sorts of ethical issues than those raised by technologies that improve quality but have little impact on quantity. Is the extension of life itself a good thing? Is it something we should seek or welcome?

On the one hand, there are circumstances in which I suspect all of us would applaud the extension of life. We have a sense that some diseases, such as childhood diabetes, cut life off or make it shorter than it "should" be. What if stem cells could be used to cure childhood diabetes, not only improving the quality of life but also permitting children diagnosed with diabetes to grow into adulthood with some confidence of being able to live a "normal" lifespan? What if we could cure or significantly ameliorate ALS, which currently kills many people in their thirties and forties? It is not hard to imagine public support for such interventions that extend life for those whose lives seem otherwise cut off "before their time." Is there a "normal" lifespan that can serve as a standard for medical intervention? Typically, that normal lifespan in the West includes living long enough not only to procreate but also raise one's children and even to see grandchildren be born and grow to young adulthood. Where lives do not hold the promise of such extension, use of stem cells to prolong life is likely to garner significant public support.

There are other circumstances as well in which stem cell interventions might be widely approved. Promising results of stem cell interventions to relieve paralysis are already being reported in both animals and human subjects. When paralysis is extensive and affects the lungs, as in the case of Christopher Reeve, it is life-threatening. Interventions to remove or ameliorate paralysis would likely extend life. Reeve served as a model for many people facing serious paralysis, and he was an outspoken advocate for stem cell research.[5] Who would not have celebrated the extension of his life? Stem cells that restored neuronal function might have spared his life, and most of us would have been very glad indeed. Thus, there are circumstances where most people would probably welcome the use of stem cell therapies that extend someone's lifespan.

However, the fact that most of us would approve or welcome extension of life in some circumstances does not necessarily make it ethically right to extend life. There are also distinctive ethical issues to be raised about the prolongation of life. Is it to be welcomed in all instances, or only in some? We may welcome it for loved individuals, but practiced on a wide scale or societal level, prolongation of life raises serious issues of justice. In the so-called First World, we already live almost *three times* as long as people in the so-called Third World (perhaps better, the "Two-Thirds World"). Better diets and easier living conditions have already extended our lives, so that a normal lifespan in the West is considerably longer than a normal lifespan in most parts of the world.[6] Stem cell technologies that prolong life are likely to increase this gap.

My mother died of congestive heart failure at age 94. She was an intelligent, gentle, dignified woman, much loved and respected by those who knew her. Stem cell technologies to repair heart and lungs might have made it possible for her to reach 100. I would have welcomed those extra years with her. Still, I must query: Is the extension of life itself a good thing? Is living to 100 a goal that we should seek? When most of the world does not live to 50, can we justify interventions that increase our lifespan from 80 years? Would it not be a global injustice to extend lifespan in the West without extending lifespan elsewhere? Indeed, those in the First World already deplete the world's resources in quantities far in excess of our population ratio. Not only do we live longer but also we are responsible for the greatest portion of the earth's degradation. To extend our lifespan would only increase this problem.

For this reason, the simple application of a measure such as "normal lifespan" is problematic. "Normal" fluctuates in accord with advances in medicine, sanitation, and wealth. "Normal" lifespans differ dramatically from culture to culture, region to region. Justice requires some redressing of that imbalance, not a perpetuation of it or even a further widening of the lifespan gap between rich and poor, with all its implications for quality of life around the globe.

For this reason, the development of stem cell technologies that extend lifespan is problematic, at least in some instances. While I would join those who seek a stem cell cure for childhood diseases that cut off life before the age of 30, once stem cell interventions are developed, they will be available for a range of diseases at different ages. Often the same technology will improve *quality* of life (e.g., by improving mobility for people with heart disease) and potentially *extend* lifespan. There is an irony here, or a paradox: the good that we do threatens also to bring about harm and injustice. This is not a tension that can easily be resolved, nor should we attempt to resolve it quickly.

Ultimately, we are confronted with the challenge of Ecclesiastes (3:2): is there a "'time to be born and a time to die"?[7] To answer a question such as this takes us outside the realm of both science and ethics and into the realm of mythology, religious belief, and fundamental metaphysical affirmations. What is the purpose of human life? What is an "excellent" human life? Is it a long life? A shorter life lived in service to others? A life long enough to complete our goals? What goals are worthy of completion? Is it sufficient to watch one's children grow up? One's grandchildren? Greatgrandchildren? If we are meant to live "abundantly," what constitutes abundance?[8] Is abundance a matter of quantity, or quality, or both? Every reader will answer these questions differently. My own answer is that there is wisdom in the affirmation that there is a time to die. Mere extension of life should not be the goal.

For these reasons, stem cell technologies have a mixed relationship to the problems of an aging society. On the one hand, many stem cell interventions hold out the promise of greatly improving the quality of life or of extending life for those who currently die "prematurely." Such improvements and extensions would no doubt be widely welcomed. On the other hand, stem cell interventions also hold out the promise of extending the lifespan and changing our sense of what is "premature" death. This consequence is much more ambiguous, and we need a great deal of public discussion of these issues as we move forward with stem cell research. At stake is our very understanding of the meaning and purpose of human life: why are we born, why do we die, and, in between birth and death, how shall we live?

NOTES

1. I follow convention here in using the term *embryonic* stem cells. However, it should be noted that such stem cells are taken from the early blastocyst and should probably more accurately be called *blastocyst stem cells.* This point was made publicly by cognitive scientist George Lakoff in an address in Fort Bragg, California, on May 27, 2005.

2. The question of public funding is the primary question addressed in the report of the President's Council on Bioethics, *Monitoring Stem Cell Research* (2004).

3. While any number of sources might be cited to support this claim, I would point to two in particular: Outka, 1987, and Walzer, 1983.

4. In *No Longer Patient: Feminist Ethics and Health Care,* Susan Sherwin (1992, 13) defines feminism as "the name given to the various theories that help reveal the multiple, gender-specific patterns of harm that constitute women's oppression." Distinguishing care-centered and power-focused feminist approaches to eth-

ics, Rosemarie Tong (1997, 49) suggests that feminist approaches center on women's "moral interests, insights, issues, and identities."

5. Reeve campaigned boldly and at considerable personal cost for stem cell research. Although he was not present in person, he recorded a brief message for the first national public conference on stem cell research, held in Berkeley, California, on June 5, 2004.

6. Ironically, our ease of living and our rich diets now threaten to be our major killers. The incidence of diabetes and other diseases associated with being overweight has risen astronomically in the United States. An ethical issue that I am not addressing here is whether access to stem cell technologies (or to any other medical intervention) should be contingent on "healthy" lifestyle choices. See Callahan, 2000.

7. Later, Ecclesiastes says, "No man has power over the wind to contain it; so no one has power over the day of his death" (8:8). And "no man knows when his hour will come" (9:12).

8. John 3:16. This passage is generally translated "eternal life." Such a translation tends to reinforce the idea that we are meant not to die, or that we are to have some form of life beyond death. For that reason, some scholars prefer the translation "abundant" life. Abundance does not necessarily imply quantity, but can refer instead to quality of life.

REFERENCES

Callahan, D., ed. 2000. *Promoting Healthy Behavior: How Much Freedom? Whose Responsibility?* Washington, DC: Georgetown University Press.

Holland, S., K. Lebacqz, and L. Zoloth, eds. 2001. *The Human Embryonic Stem Cell Debate* Cambridge, MA: MIT Press.

Lanza, R, and N. Rosenthal. 2004. The stem cell challenge. *Scientific American* 290:92–99.

Outka, G. 1987. Social justice and equal access to health care. In *On Moral Medicine: Theological Perspectives in Medical Ethics,* ed. Stephen E. Lammers and Allen Verhey. Grand Rapids, MI: Wm. B. Eerdmans.

President's Council on Bioethics. 2004. *Monitoring Stem Cell Research.* Washington, DC: President's Council on Bioethics.

Sherwin, S. 1992. *No Longer Patient: Feminist Ethics and Health Care.* Philadelphia: Temple University Press.

Snow, N., ed. 2003. *Stem Cell Research: New Frontiers in Science and Ethics.* South Bend, IN: University of Notre Dame Press.

Tong, R. 1997. *Feminist Approaches to Bioethics: Theoretical Reflections and Practical Applications.* Boulder, CO: Westview Press.

Walzer, M. 1983. *Spheres of Justice: A Defense of Pluralism and Equality.* New York: Basic Books.

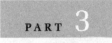

PART 3

CENTENARIANS

CHAPTER 8

Centenarians and Genetics

THOMAS T. PERLS, M.D., M.P.H.

Improvements in public health measures in the twentieth century resulted in a transformation in the age distribution of the population of industrialized nations. There was a 60 percent increase in average life expectancy, up from 46 years in 1900 to 77 years today (Centers for Disease Control and Prevention, 2005). This increase can be traced to numerous factors, including water supply safety, better living and work conditions, the development of health interventions such as antibiotics, and better treatment of age-related illnesses such as hypertension and heart disease. As a result, many more people who would have otherwise died as children and in middle age now have the opportunity to achieve the lifespans that their environment and genetic makeup will allow. Centenarians have become the fastest growing age group, in part because there were relatively few of them just twenty years ago. Over the next three decades, the aged population in the United States will increase to the point that there will be as many people over the age of 65 as there are under the age of 20. The impact of the baby-boomers is clearly demonstrated by the projected sudden increase in the age 65+ group in 2010 and the age 85+ group in 2030 (He et al., 2005).

While the increase in average life expectancy over the past century reflects the overall improvement in public health, disturbing trends have emerged in children, women, and minority groups. Olshansky and colleagues (2005) have pointed out that increasing rates of obesity, particularly among children, are leading to increased rates of age-related illnesses that could result in a deceleration in survival rates. Hispanics experience disproportionate rates of diabetes mellitus along with resulting morbidities such as blindness, congestive heart failure, amputations, and kidney failure. While rates of smoking are declining among white men, this is not the case among women, teenagers, or minorities. The substantial disparity in mortality rates between Caucasians and African Americans over age 20 could be nearly obviated if we were much more effective in detecting and treating hypertension in the latter group (Graham et al., 2006).

Centenarians

The growing population of centenarians is of particular interest to a discussion of aging, technology, and genetics. In the United States, approximately 1 in 100,000 persons was a centenarian at the turn of the twentieth century, and this figure has now grown to 1.2 in 10,000. Worldwide, among industrialized countries, the number of centenarians is increasing at the rate of about 8 percent per year (Vaupel et al., 1998).

In most populations, 85 percent of centenarians are women. Though women are more likely to achieve exceptional longevity than men, male centenarians have better functional status, at least in some populations. One explanation for this may be that men must be in excellent health to achieve such extreme old age (Perls, 1998). Women, on the other hand, may be better adept at living with age-associated illnesses, and thus they can achieve exceptional old age even with significant chronic disability. These observations might indicate a demographic crossover in which women are better off than men in younger old age and men, although fewer in number, are functionally better off in extreme old age.

What Life Expectancy and Lifespan Are We Built For?

People vary a great deal in terms of how they age. Some seem to age relatively quickly and develop age-related illnesses such as heart disease or stroke in their forties and fifties, while others appear to age slowly and develop age-related illnesses only toward the end of very long lives. Within these two extremes are the majority of people who, at least in industrialized nations, have an average life expectancy in their late seventies. Much of the variation around this average appears to be due to differences in genetics, environment, behavior, and luck. The advantages of good health habits are highlighted by the case of the Seventh Day Adventists, who appear to be capable of achieving average survival into their late eighties (Fraser and Shavlik, 2001). The behavioral traits that lead to such a survival advantage are regular exercise, a frugal vegetarian diet, not smoking, and perhaps the advantages of religious faith in managing stress.

Twin studies have estimated the genetic component of life expectancy to range between 25 and 30 percent (McGue et al., 1993). These twin studies do not, however, estimate the heritability of living to extreme old age, because the oldest subjects in these studies are only octogenarians. Centenarians, who live an additional 15 to 20 years beyond average life expectancy, may require an additional genetic advantage, particularly if they maintain high cognitive function at very old age (McClearn et al., 1997).

Perls and colleagues (2002) analyzed the pedigrees of 444 families in the United States that included 2,092 siblings of centenarians. Survival was compared with the 1900 birth cohort survival data from the U.S. Social Security Administration. Female siblings had death rates at all ages that were about one-half the national level; male siblings had a similar advantage at most ages, though it diminished somewhat during adolescence and young adulthood. The siblings had an average age of death of 76.7 for females and 70.4 for males compared with 58.3 and 51.5 for the general population born around the same time. Even after accounting for race and education, the net survival advantage of siblings of centenarians was found to be 16 to 17 years greater than the general population. Relative survival probabilities (RSP) for these siblings increased markedly at older ages, reflecting the cumulative effect of their mortality advantage throughout life. Compared with the U.S. 1900 birth cohort, male siblings of centenarians were 17 times as likely to attain age 100 themselves, while female siblings were 8.2 times as likely.

The analysis of death rates indicates that the siblings' mortality advantage does not increase as they get older. Rather, their relative probability of survival is a cumulative measure and reflects their life-long advantage over the general population born about the same time. Taken together, these data support the hypothesis that centenarians and their family members have genetic variations in common that are important to achieving exceptional longevity.

Because mortality rates of different groups (e.g., differing by gender, race, education, physical activity, socioeconomic status) converge at very old age, the difference in survival among these groups is surprising. The substantially higher RSP values for men at older ages might reflect the fact that male disease-specific mortality is significantly higher than for females at these older ages and thus the males experience a greater relative advantage from beneficial genotypes compared with women. Another possibility could be that a more uncommon combination of genetic and environmental factors is required for men to achieve extreme age compared with women. Either possibility could explain why men comprise only 15 percent of centenarians.

Richard Cutler (1975), in what is now a classic paper in gerontology, proposed that persons who achieve extreme old age do so in part because they have genetic variations that affect the basic mechanisms of aging and that result in a uniform decreased susceptibility to age-associated diseases. Persons who achieve extreme old age probably lack many of the variations ("disease genes") that substantially increase risk for premature death by predisposing persons to fatal diseases. More controversial is the idea that genetic variations might confer protection against the basic mechanisms of aging or age-related illnesses (the "longevity-enabling genes"). Centenarians may be rare because a complex set of environmental and genetic variables must coexist for such survival to occur.

The fact that siblings maintain only half the mortality risk of their birth cohort from age 20 to extreme age suggests a multifactorial model for achieving exceptional longevity. For example, sociodemographic advantages may impact survival at younger ages, while genetic advantages may emerge as persons move from old age to extreme old age. Undoubtedly, exceptional longevity is much more complicated, with temporally overlapping roles for single genetic, polygenic, environmental, and stochastic components. Such a scenario would be consistent with a "threshold model," where predisposition for exceptional longevity can be measured on a quantitative scale. Such a model, proposed by Falconer (1965), predicts that the proportion of affected relatives will be highest among the most severely affected individuals. Examples of disease phenotypes fitting the threshold model are early-onset breast cancer or Alzheimer disease (AD), where relatives of patients who develop these diseases at unusually young ages are themselves at increased risk or liability. Thus, a 108-year-old person's "liability" or predisposition for exceptional longevity is further beyond the threshold in comparison with someone more mildly affected (e.g., a person who died at age 99 years). The higher RSP of male siblings of centenarians compared with female siblings may mean that males carry a higher liability for the trait given the presence of the requisite traits. The threshold model predicts that if a multifactorial trait is more frequent in one sex (as is the case with exceptional longevity, which is predominantly represented by females), the liability will be higher for relatives of the less "susceptible" sex (males, in the case of exceptional longevity) (Farrer and Cupples, 1998). The model also predicts that the risk for exceptional longevity will be sharply lower for second-degree relatives compared with first-degree relatives. If this model holds true for exceptional longevity, it suggests that (1) the older the subject, the more power for discovering traits predisposing for exceptional longevity; and (2) there are gender-related differences in both relatives and probands in their "liability" for exceptional longevity.

Genes Predisposing to Exceptional Longevity

The discovery of genetic variations that explain even 5–10 percent of the variation in survival to extreme old age could yield important clues about the cellular and biochemical mechanisms that affect basic mechanisms of aging and susceptibility to age-associated diseases. Until recently, only one genetic variation had been reproducibly associated with exceptional longevity. Schachter and colleagues (1994) from the French Centenarian Study noted that the apolipoprotein E e4 allele becomes markedly less frequent with advancing age. One of its counterparts, the e2 allele, becomes more frequent with advancing age in Caucasians (Rebeck et al., 1994).

Nir Barzilai and colleagues studying Ashkenazi Jewish centenarians and their families investigated a cardiovascular pathway and gene that is differentially associated with centenarians and controls who were spouses of the children of centenarians. Barzilai and colleagues (2003) also noted that high-density lipoprotein (HDL) and low-density lipoprotein (LDL) particles were significantly larger among the centenarians and their off-spring, and that particle size also differentiated between subjects with and without cardiovascular disease, hypertension, and metabolic syndrome. In a candidate-gene approach, the researchers then searched the literature for genes that affect HDL and LDL particle size, and hepatic lipase and cholesteryl ester transfer protein (CETP) emerged as candidates. Compared with a control group representative of the general population, centenarians themselves were three times as likely, and their offspring were twice as likely, to have a specific CETP gene variant.

Achieving Very Old Age: Good or Bad News?

Some have contended that survival to exceptional old age is inevitably accompanied by co-morbidities and prolonged disability (Gruenberg, 1977; Verghese et al., 2003). In contrast, the "compression of morbidity hypothesis," introduced in 1980, optimistically suggests that at very old ages, the prevalence of co-morbidities and disability will be compressed toward the end of life, thus reducing the overall time of health decline (Fries, 1980). Vita and colleagues (1998), in their more than 40-year longitudinal study of university alumni, found that people with the best health habits (not smoking, regular physical activity, normal body mass index) lived longer and compressed the number of years lived with disability over a shorter period of time at the end of life. Ferrucci and colleagues (1999), in a population-based study, similarly found that nonsmokers with high levels of physical activity had a longer disability-free life expectancy compared with physically inactive smokers.

One would expect that the phenomenon of compression of morbidity and disability would be most apparent among centenarians who truly do approach the limits of lifespan, and there is some evidence to support this. Morbidity was compressed beyond the age of 80 years in 60 percent of New England Centenarian Study subjects (Evert et al., 2003). When examining only the most lethal diseases of older people, such as heart disease, non-skin cancer, and stroke, 87 percent of males and 83 percent of females delayed or escaped these diseases altogether.

The degree of disability plays an important role in determining whether centenarians compress mortality. In the Swedish Centenarian Study, 25 percent of the subjects lived in their own home, 37 percent in assisted living, and 38 percent in nursing homes. In the New England Centenarian Study, the proportions were similar, with approximately 15 percent living independently in their own homes, 35 percent living with family or in assisted living, and 50 percent living in nursing homes. While the majority of centenarians experience some functional disability, this disability also appears to be compressed toward the end of life. In the New England Centenarian Study's population-based sample, 90 percent of centenarians were independently functioning at the mean age of 92 years (Hitt et al., 1999). In particular, most subjects experienced a decline in their cognitive function only in the last three to five years of their lives. With this work in mind, we have proposed an empowering perspective of aging—that is, "The older you get, the healthier you've been," as opposed to the inherent ageism of the more common statement, "The older you get, the sicker you get."

However, centenarians do not always escape morbidity. In the New England Centenarian Study, 24 percent of male centenarians and 43 percent of female centenarians fell into a "survivor" category, in which they survived with one or more major age-related illnesses for 20 or more years. The delay in disability despite a long history of illness might be due to "resilience," representing increased functional reserve and/or adaptive capacity. The ramifications of these findings are that among older people, morbidity and disability do not always go hand in hand and that a third phenomenon, resilience, must be considered. Eventually, being able to quantify this resilience and to understand its underlying mechanisms could lead to better prognostication and perhaps even therapies.

Regarding cognitive function in exceptional old age, the population-based Heidelberg Centenarian Study reported that about 50 percent of centenarians demonstrated moderate to severe cognitive impairment, and about 25 percent were found to be cognitively intact (Kliegel, Moor, and Rott, 2004). These proportions are approximately the same as the cognitive function studies reported by the Danish, Swedish, Georgia, and New England Centenarian Studies, which indicated that about 70 percent of centenarians were cognitively impaired and 30 percent were cognitively intact (Andersen-Ranberg, Vasegaard, and Jeune, 2001; Hagberg et al., 2001; Silver, Jilinskaia, and Perls, 2001). With strict criteria for no evidence of cognitive impairment, about 12–15 percent of centenarians show no evidence of impairment.

Several contenarian studies conducted neuropsychological testing followed by postmortem neuropathological studies, which have led to several interesting observations. A number of cases have been described of centenarians who were cognitively intact near the time of death and at autopsy were found to have no evidence of neuropathology including neurofibrillary tangles and neuritic plaques—pathological markers once thought to be inevitable consequences of aging and that are the pathological hallmarks of Alzheimer disease (Silver et al., 1998). These cases might be considered examples of disease-free aging, and they support the notion that for some people, neuropathology is not an inevitable consequence of aging, and that aging alone is not necessarily associated with the presence of pathology.

Of additional interest has been the observation by some researchers that the frequencies of various dementia types are different among people who were nonagenarians or older compared with younger cohorts. While AD is generally accepted as the most common cause for dementia among persons who survive to the sixth, seventh, and eighth decades, the Danish Centenarian Study reported that 50 percent of the dementia cases among centenarians were due to vascular disease (Andersen-Ranberg, Vasegaard, and Jeune, 2001). An autopsy series of 13 Japanese centenarians who were normal or only mildly impaired revealed vascular but not AD pathology (Itoh et al., 1998). It is likely that rare causes of dementia become more common among centenarians because people who are prone to develop AD die at younger ages, and survivors will clinically express other neurodegenerative illnesses such as vascular dementia, Pick disease, and Lewy body disease.

Genetics and Lifespan: Does It Matter?

Human longevity-enabling genes are likely to influence aging at its most basic levels, thus affecting a broad spectrum of genetic and cellular pathways synchronously. The centenarian genome also holds some promise for ferreting out genes that protect against common diseases or reduce the mortality of common diseases. For example, researchers are in the early stages of understanding differential gene expression in models known to slow the aging process, such as caloric restriction. Studies of such models might uncover longevity-enabling genes that are targets for the creation of drugs that allow persons to become more "centenarianlike" by maximizing the period of their lives spent in good health.

It should be noted, however, that the vast majority of the increases in average life expectancy that we have experienced over the past century are attributable to major changes in public health. Further interventions along these lines, such as strategies to decrease obesity and smoking, decrease the impact of stress, and increase healthy diets and daily exercise will still have the greatest impact on any potential increase in average life expectancy in the foreseeable future.

ACKNOWLEDGMENTS

This work is supported by the National Institute on Aging (U01-AG-023755, K24 AG25727).

REFERENCES

Andersen-Ranberg, K., L. Vasegaard, and B. Jeune. 2001. Dementia is not inevitable: A population-based study of Danish centenarians. *Journals of Gerontology Series B: Psychological Sciences and Social Sciences* 56:P152–59.

Barzilai N. A. G., C. Schechter, E. J. Schaefer, A. L. Cupples, R. Lipton, S. Cheng, and A. R. Shuldiner. 2003. Unique lipoprotein phenotype and genotype in humans with exceptional longevity. *Journal of the American Medical Association* 290:2030–40.

Centers for Disease Control and Prevention. 2005. National Center for Health Statistics, *Health, United States, 2005,* figure 26.

Cutler, R. 1975. Evolution of human longevity and the genetic complexity govern ing aging rate. *Proceedings of the National Academy of Sciences of the United States of America* 72:4664–68.

Evert, J., E. Lawler, H. Bogan, and T. Perls. 2003. Morbidity profiles of centenarians: Survivors, delayers, and escapers. *Journals of Gerontology Series A: Biological Sciences and Medical Sciences* 58:M232–37.

Falconer, D. 1965. The inheritance and liability to certain disease estimated from the incidence among relatives. *Annals of Human Genetics* 29:51–76.

Farrer, L., and A. Cupples. 1998. Determining the genetic component of a disease. In *Approaches to Gene Mapping in Complex Human Diseases,* ed. J. Haines and M. A. Pericak-Vance. New York: Wiley-Liss.

Ferrucci, L., G. Izmirlian, S. Leveille, C. L. Phillips, M. C. Corti, D. B. Brock, et al. 1999. Smoking, physical activity, and active life expectancy. *American Journal of Epidemiology* 140:645–55.

Fraser, G. E., and D. J. Shavlik. 2001. Ten years of life: Is it a matter of choice? *Archives of Internal Medicine* 161:1645–52.

Fries, J. F. 1980. Aging, natural death, and the compression of morbidity. *New England Journal of Medicine* 303:130–35.

Graham, G. N., B. Leath, K. Payne, M. Guendelman, G.Reynolds, S. Kim, et al. 2006. Perceived versus actual risk for hypertension and diabetes in the African American community. *Health Promotion Practice* 7:34–46.

Gruenberg, E. 1977. The failure of success. *Milbank Memorial Fund Quarterly* 5:3–34.

Hagberg B., B. B. Alfredson, L. W. Poon, and A. Homma. 2001. Cognitive function-ing in centenarians: A coordinated analysis of results from three countries. *Journals of Gerontology Series B: Psychological Sciences and Social Sciences* 56:P141–51.

He, W., M. Sengupta, V. A. Velkoff, and K. A. DeBarros, 2005. 65+ in the United States, 2005. U.S. Department of Health and Human Services. Retrieved from www.census.gov/prod/2006pubs/p23–209.pdf, February 12, 2007.

Hitt, R., Y. Young-Xu, M. Silver, and T. Perls. 1999. Centenarians: The older you get, the healthier you have been. *Lancet* 354:652.

Itoh, Y., M. Yamada, N. Suematsu, M. Matsushita, and E. Otomo. 1998. An immu-nohistochemical study of centenarian brains: A comparison. *Journal of Neuro-logical Science* 157:73–81.

Kliegel M., C. Moor, and C. Rott. 2004. Cognitive status and development in the oldest old: A longitudinal analysis from the Heidelberg Centenarian Study. *Archives of Gerontology and Geriatrics* 39:143–56.

McClearn, G. E., B. Johansson, S. Berg , N. L. Pedersen, F. Ahern, S. A. Petrill, and R. Plomin. 1997. Substantial genetic influence on cognitive abilities in twins 80 or more years old. *Science* 276:1560–63.

McGue, M., J. W. Vaupel, N. Holm, and B. Harvald. 1993. Longevity is moderately heritable in a sample of Danish twins born 1870–1880. *Journal of Gerontology* 48:B237–44.

Olshansky, S. J., D. J. Passaro, R. C. Hershow, J. Layden , B. A. Carnes, J. Brody, et al. 2005. A potential decline in life expectancy in the United States in the 21st century. *New England Journal of Medicine* 352:1138–45.

Perls, T., and R. Fretts. 1998. Why women live longer than men. *Scientific Ameri-can Presents,* 100–107.

Perls, T. T., J. Wilmoth, R. Levenson, M. Drinkwater, M. Cohen, H. Bogan, et al. 2002. Life-long sustained mortality advantage of siblings of centenarians. *Pro-ceedings of the National Academy of Sciences of the United States of America* 99:8442–47.

Rebeck, G. W., T. T. Perls, H. L. West, P. Sodhi, L. A. Lipsitz, and B. T. Hyman. 1994. Reduced apolipoprotein epsilon 4 allele frequency in the oldest old Alzheimer's patients and cognitively normal individuals. *Neurology* 44:1513–16.

Schachter, F., L. Faure-Delanef, F. Guenot, H. Rouger, P. Froguel, L. Lesueur-Ginot, et al. 1994. Genetic associations with human longevity at the APOE and ACE loci. *Nature Genetics* 6(1):29–32.

Silver, M., K. Newell, B. Hyman, J. Growdon, E. T. Hedley-Whyte, and T. Perls. 1998. Unraveling the mystery of cognitive changes in old age: Correlation of neuropsychological evaluation with neuropathological findings in the extreme old. *International Psychogeriatrics* 10(1):25–41.

Silver, M. H., E. Jilinskaia, and T. T. Perls. 2001. Cognitive functional status of age-confirmed centenarians in a population-based study. *Journals of Gerontology, Series B: Psychological Sciences and Social Sciences* 56:P134–40.

Vaupel, J. W., J. R. Carey, K. Christensen, T. E. Johnson, A. I. Yashin, A. N. V. Holm, et al. 1998. Biodemographic trajectories of longevity. *Science* 280:855–60.

Verghese, J., R. B. Lipton, M. J. Katz, C. B. Hall, C. A. Derby, G. Kuslansky, et al. 2003. Leisure activities and the risk of dementia in the elderly. *New England Journal of Medicine* 348:2508–16.

Vita, A. J., R. B. Terry, H. B. Hubert, and J. F. Fries. 1998. Aging, health risks, and cumulative disability. *New England Journal of Medicine* 338:1035–41.

CHAPTER 9

What Can We Learn from Centenarians?

LEONARD W. POON, PH.D.

Malcolm Cowley, an essayist, poet, and former editor of the *New Republic* magazine, wrote, "To enter the country of old age is a new experience, different from what you supposed it to be. Nobody, man or woman, knows the country until he has lived in it and has taken out his citizenship papers" (1991, 3). According to Mr. Cowley, I don't have any business writing about being a centenarian. In fact, few individuals could claim to live to 100 and talk legitimately about the experiences of very old age. In my studies of centenarians since 1988, I began by identifying attributes of centenarians that are different from those with little chance of becoming centenarians (those who are in their eighties and sixties). It is important to note the potential confounding of cohort effects in this type of research as well as the difficulty of isolating survival factors in aging and special populations. Although it seems that some survival characteristics could be identified, I marveled at the large individual differences among the survivors and the many paths they could employ to achieve their longevity.

Who Are the Centenarians?

The older segments of our population are increasing in number at faster rates than the rest of the population, and the 65-and-older population is growing much more rapidly compared with the 65-and-younger segments (Himes, 2002). Among the 65+ population, the 100+ segment is the fastest growing. One can observe over the last century that the oldest of our population increased from a negligible number to an appreciable portion of our population. In the 2000 census, the number of centenarians was counted as 50,454 nationwide (1,135 in my home state of Georgia). At present, most industrialized countries in the world have about 1 centenarian per 10,000 of their population, and the trend is toward 1 in 5,000. As one can easily project, the reality of this rapid increase has significant health care, caregiving, economic, social, family, and interpersonal implications.

How Are Centenarians Different from Their Birth Cohorts?

It may be difficult for many to fathom and appreciate the experiences of an individual who has lived 100 years. Let us examine the experiences of a centenarian who was born at the turn of the twentieth century. The average lifespan of Americans at 1900 was about 50 years, 48.5 years for males and 51 for females. From this perspective, a centenarian born in 1900 would have lived two lifetimes compared with his birth cohort. This is perhaps the one single factor that makes a centenarian special and unique. I, for one, would have a difficult time imagining that some of my birth cohort could live twice as long as me.

When this centenarian was born in 1900, Orville and Wilbur Wright had not yet built their first airplane, and Einstein had not yet published his theory of relativity. St. Louis was the host city for the World's Fair, and the ice cream cone was being introduced. The first radio transmission was broadcast at about that time, and the Model T Ford was introduced. This individual would have experienced World War 1 as a teenager in 1914. When this individual was in his twenties, the Constitution was amended to grant suffrage to women, Charles Lindbergh piloted the *Spirit of St. Louis* on the first nonstop transatlantic flight, and Americans watched the first long-distance television broadcast.

This centenarian would have experienced a long list of "firsts" during the formative years. Imagine the excitement of watching an automobile drive by, or hearing sound and seeing pictures transmitted to one's home. When this centenarian was 29 years of age, the Great Depression would have begun. This would be a profound experience for a young person at the prime of life. While perhaps too old for military service in World War II, this centenarian and his birth cohorts would have experienced two world wars by 40 years of age.

While an average person born in 1900 would have lived to about 1950, this future centenarian would have lived another 50 years and continued to experience major shifts such as the cultural upheavals of the 1960s, the assassination of John F. Kennedy in 1963, the first landing of men on the moon in 1969, the discovery and spread of the AIDS virus in the 1980s, the U.S. space shuttle *Challenger* explosion in 1986, and the breakup of the Soviet Union in 1990. Finally, after his one-hundredth birthday, this centenarian would have shared the nation's horror at a terrorist attack on September 11, 2001.

While we do know that an individual's experiences can demonstrably influence perception, motivation, behavior, and even personality and coping styles, there is limited information on the impact of such lifelong experiences upon the perceptions and behaviors of centenarians. This, I believe, is a critical research area to better understand individual and cohort differences at the end stage of life.

How Are Centenarians Different from 80- and 60-Year-Old Cohorts?

Our study of centenarians began in 1988 as an attempt to answer the question of how centenarians differ from younger cohorts. It is important to note that findings from a cross-sectional study comparing centenarians with younger cohorts could potentially be confounded by cohort effects. That is, a person born in 1900 would have significantly different experiences than those born in 1920 and 1940, and these cohort effects could be misinterpreted as effects related to survival. Indeed, one of the difficulties in centenarian research is the selection of control groups. Who could or should be compared with centenarians to demonstrate their unique characteristics? There are potentially three approaches to this problem. The first is to start with middle-aged adults and follow them longitudinally, examining the impact and life course of those who are able to reach advanced ages compared with those who do not. This approach is impractical because the time to completion of such a study would be many decades. While some existing adult longitudinal studies could in time provide some answers to the questions, most of these are not large enough to ultimately yield a sufficient number of centenarians to study.

A second solution would be to compare centenarian survivors with groups of people whose survival probability to 100 is very small. This is the strategy we employed in our first centenarian study (1988–1992), funded by the National Institute of Mental Health, wherein we compared 100-, 80-, and 60-year-old cohorts (Poon et al., 1992). The probability that a 60- or 80-year-old will survive to the age of 100 is 1 percent and 0.5 percent, respectively, so these groups can, to some extent, be construed as "future noncentenarians." Our first study attempted to compare centenarians with noncentenarians. Following these populations over time adds a longitudinal component to the comparison, and this strategy was employed in our second study of centenarians (1992–1998), again funded by the National Institute of Mental Health.

A third approach is to perform a population-based study of centenarians, examining the individual characteristics of the entire distribution of centenarians varying in genetic makeup, health, pathologies, cognitive abilities, functions, dependencies, and support systems. In this manner the different pathways to centenarian survival could be compared and described. This is the strategy we are currently using in a project (2001–2007) that is in the third year of funding from the National Institute on Aging.

How are centenarians different from their younger cohorts? While results of our current study are pending, the remainder of this chapter summarizes results from the first two studies of centenarians in Georgia.

Figure 9.1 outlines the hypothetical model and hypotheses in terms of direct and indirect influences that make up potential predictors to long-term survival. The overall goal of our early centenarian studies was to compare and contrast factors leading to "successful adaptation" of community-dwelling and cognitively intact centenarians, octogenarians, and sexagenarians. Successful adaptation in this model was defined as a perception of high morale and life satisfaction. From this perspective, we have included a host of predictors that could either directly or indirectly contribute to these outcomes. These predictors are family longevity, envi-

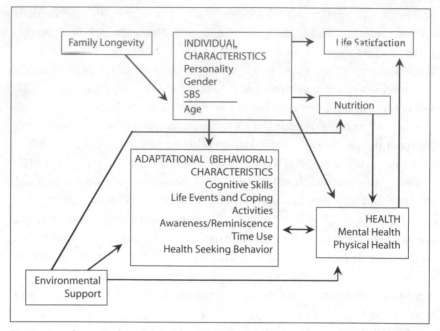

Figure 9.1. Theoretical model and hypotheses of the Georgia Centenarian Study.
Source: Poon, L. W. et al. 1992. The Georgia Centenarian Study. *International Journal of Aging and Human Development* 34 (1):6. Reprinted with permission, Baywood Publishing Company, Inc.

ronmental support, individual characteristics, adaptation characteristics, nutrition, and physical and mental health. We asked three sets of questions: (1) How are community-dwelling and cognitively intact centenarians different in these predictors and outcome characteristics compared with younger cohorts? (2) How do these predictors directly and indirectly influence morale and life satisfaction among the three cohorts? (3) How well can the hypothetical model predict morale and life satisfaction?

It is important to note that this study of survival and adaptation focuses on community-dwelling and cognitively intact centenarians, octogenarians, and sexagenarians. From this perspective, the findings are not representative of or generalizable to the centenarians at large. Participants who met inclusion criteria were recruited from throughout the state of Georgia, and 78 centenarians, 93 octogenarians, and 91 sexagenarians participated. Women accounted for 76 percent, 67 percent, and 58 percent of the three respective age groups, and these proportions were similar to the age-appropriate gender distributions in the Georgia population. Further, race distributions were also similar to the population in their respective age groups in Georgia (67%, 77%, and 72% Caucasians, respectively).

We found six principal characteristics that differentiated centenarians from the two younger cohorts.

Health and health habits. Consistent with the findings from the Alameda County Study (Breslow and Breslow, 1993) and the Harvard College Alumni Study (Paffenbarger et al., 1994), the Georgia centenarians tended to practice health habits that were found to prolong life (Nickols-Richardson et al., 1996). That is, few smoked, were obese, or consumed excessive alcohol. They remained active throughout life and ate breakfast on a regular basis. Compared with cohorts in their sixties and eighties, centenarians tended to escape contracting chronic diseases during their lifetime.

Dietary habits. With few exceptions, the intake of most nutrients was similar among 60-, 80-, and 100-year-old community-dwelling groups (Fischer et al., 1995; Williams et al., 1995; Johnson et al., 1992). Centenarians consumed about 20–30 percent more carotenoids and vitamin A from foods, consumed breakfast regularly and avoided fluctuations in body weight, and tended to consume more whole milk, less 2 percent milk and yogurt, and were less likely to avoid dietary cholesterol (reflecting the Southern diet of the early 1900s). It is important to note that centenarians tended to consume all foods in moderation.

Cognition and intelligence. Comparing cognitively intact centenarians with younger cohorts, centenarians showed poorer performances in most cognitive functions except for everyday problem-solving tasks (Holtsberg et al., 1995; Poon et al., 1992). The magnitudes of age differences were smaller in crystallized intelligence than in fluid intelligence. Education was shown to have a strong positive effect that mitigated the level of performance differences between subjects, especially centenarians. When centenarians used their everyday experiences in problem solving, their performances were found to be similar to the younger cohorts (Poon et al., 1992). Regression models suggested that cognition accounted for about 20 percent of the variance in Instrumental Activities of Daily Living (IADL) for all subjects. When functional and mental health, as well as social and economic resources, was included in the regression equation, the amount of IADL variance that could be predicted increased to 37 percent. These findings show that cognition, health, and resources are all important predictors of everyday functions.

Personality and coping styles. Centenarians were more dominant, suspicious, practical, and relaxed than those in their sixties and eighties (Martin et al., 1992). Centenarians were less likely to use active behavioral coping but were more likely to use cognitive coping behaviors when compared with octogenarians (Martin et al., 1992). Centenarians were more likely to acknowledge problems than those in other age groups, and they were less likely to seek social support as a coping strategy for their problems.

Support systems. Community-dwelling centenarians reported fewer potential visitors. They were less likely to talk on the telephone or have a spouse as a primary caregiver but more likely to have their children as caregivers and to receive help with food and meal preparation from family and friends (Martin et al., 1996). However, they were just as likely as those in their sixties and eighties to have someone help them if they were sick or disabled, to have a confidante, and to have daily visitors.

Mental health. Compared with younger community-dwelling cohorts, centenarians tended to report more somatic but not emotional symptoms. Although centenarians were found to have a higher level of depression, measured by the Geriatric Depression Scale (Yesavage et al., 1983), as compared with younger cohorts, no clinical depression was found among the sample of community-dwelling centenarians. A comment on our findings on race difference is offered here. African-American centenarians were found to have significantly higher levels of depression and poorer self-perceived health than their Caucasian counterparts. However, when education and income were taken into account, differences in self-perceived health were eliminated, and differences in mental health decreased but remained significant (Kim et al., 1998). This was found for all three age groups. This finding shows that concomitant measures such as education, socioeconomic background, and mental health are important and could influence survivorship and quality of life of the oldest old.

Can We Predict Days of Survival after 100 Years?

As noted earlier, some of the characteristics noted to differentiate centenarian survivors from younger controls could be due to cohort effects. We therefore asked which variables, if any, could predict days of survival after an individual attained the age of 100. If the variables associated with extended survival among the centenarians themselves are the same as the variables associated with centenarian survival in comparison with younger cohorts, this would add confidence to the inferences made using the younger cohort.

We conducted an analysis of survival among 137 centenarians (Poon et al., 2000). At the time of initial testing, the participants' average age was 100.8 years. The outcome variable of interest was days of survival after reaching the one-hundredth birthday. Predictor variables include demographic variables, family longevity, physical health measures, functional health variables, cognitive status variables, and psychological self-report. Our analyses revealed that five clusters of variables were viable predictors of days of survival among centenarians: gender, family longevity, income and social support, anthropometrics, and cognition.

1. On average, women survived 1,020 days after attaining 100 years, while men survived an average of 781 days. This gender difference in survival was not significant after two years but became significant after three years.
2. The age of death of the centenarian's father's was positively associated with the days of survival of centenarians. No effect was found for mother's age of death.
3. Three social support factors were associated with increased survival among centenarians. They were talking on the phone, having someone to help, and having a caregiver.
4. Three anthropometric measures were found to correlate positively to survival: triceps skinfold (an index of body fat), body mass index, and waist-to-hip ratio.
5. Higher levels of cognitive ability after age 100 were positively associated with longer length of survival.

Our data show that there are indeed quantifiable predictors that could reliably predict days of survivorship after 100 years. The implications of this finding are discussed in the next section.

What Lessons Can We Learn from Centenarians?

The notion that aging and death could be postponed or even avoided has existed throughout human history. The ancient Greeks, for example, invented the myth of the Hyperboreans, a perpetually youthful people who lived in a land of sunshine and abundance. The explorer Ponce de Leon challenged our imagination by attempting to locate the fountain of youth. Likewise, the English novelist James Hilton wrote of the discovery of Shangri-La, the land of eternal youth. The challenge to prolong life is as in vogue today as at any time in human history. Are there specific secrets that could unlock the puzzle?

As a centenarian researcher, I am bombarded with these questions weekly from the media. I am certain that my fellow centenarian researchers in the United States and elsewhere can share similar experiences. What are the secrets to delayed mortality? Can the centenarians themselves reveal such secrets? Could the discovery of new scientific breakthroughs in advanced longevity be just around the corner?

After 17 years of studying centenarians, I am still unable to provide definitive answers. Indeed, the more I study factors that can contribute to longevity, the more I think about the impact of the human spirit and of human choices as determinant of longevity. While biological and genetic factors are clearly important, we still do not understand how they may interact with environmental and intra-individual contributions to determine and prolong life.

It has been estimated that heredity contributes about 30 percent toward the extraordinary longevity of centenarians. If this is true, it would mean that about 70 percent of extreme longevity could be environmentally based (nutrition, living conditions, coping, attitudes, health promotion and maintenance, reduction of risk taking behaviors, etc.). In the Georgia Centenarian Study survival analyses of longevity after the first 100 years, among the five identified predictors, two are genetically based (gender and family longevity) and three are environmentally based (social support, sufficient nourishment, and cognition). From this perspective, human attitudes and choices may underlie the secrets of longevity.

If healthy lifestyle practices are associated with longer lives, then why do some people who practice healthy lifestyles fail to live beyond average lifespans? Further, why do some who tend not to subscribe to these practices (such as lifelong smokers) live much longer than the average? From the data we have acquired so far from the Georgia Centenarian Study, it is my belief that there are many paths to longevity as evidenced by the distribution of factors that accounted for the total longevity variance. For some centenarians, heredity seems to exert a significant influence given the large number of long-lived relatives in their family tree. Other centenarians, who do not have any long-lived relatives, may possess personality and coping styles that tend to facilitate long lives. For others, their superior problem solving and intellectual abilities seem to be the dominating contributors. Also, for some centenarians there may not be any distinguishable attributes that seem to stand out.

When we asked our centenarians for their formula for longevity, we received a vast variety of responses. Some provided a specific formula, such as clean living, work ethic, religion, diligence, eating habits, and so on. Others noted perhaps the most telling philosophy of all: that they lived one day at a time, and pretty soon they were centenarians.

REFERENCES

Breslow, L., and N. Breslow. 1993. Health practices and disability: Some evidence from Alameda County. *Preventive Medicine* 22(1):86–95.

Cowley, M. 1991. From the view from 80. In *Songs of Experience: An Anthology of Literature on Growing Old,* ed. M. Fowler and P. McCutcheon. Pp. 8–9. New York: Ballantine.

Fischer, J. C., M. A. Johnson, L. W. Poon, and P. Martin. 1995. Dairy product intake of the oldest old. *Journal of the American Dietetics Association* 95:918–21.

Johnson, M. A., M. A. Brown, L. W. Poon, P. Martin, and G. M. Clayton. 1992. Nutritional patterns of centenarians. *International Journal of Aging and Human Development* 34(1):57–76.

Himes, C. L. 2002. Elderly Americans. *Population Bulletin* 56(4):4.

Holtsberg, P. A., L. W. Poon, C. A. Noble, and P. Martin. 1995. Mini-Mental State Exam status of community-dwelling cognitively intact centenarians. *International Psychogeriatrics* 7:417–27.

Kim, J., M. H. Bramlett, L. K. Wright, and L. W. Poon. 1998. Racial differences in health status and factors that influence health behaviors in older adults. *Nursing Research* 47:243–50.

Martin, P., L. W. Poon, G. M. Clayton, H. S. Lee, J. S. Fulks, and M. A. Johnson. 1992. Personality, life events, and coping in the oldest old. *International Journal of Aging and Human Development* 34(special issue 1):19–30.

Martin, P., L. W. Poon, E. Kim, and M. A. Johnson. 1996. Social and psychological resources of the oldest old. *Experimental Aging Research* 22:121–39.

Nickols-Richardson, S. M., M. A. Johnson, L. W. Poon, and P. Martin. 1996. Demographic predictors of nutritional risk in elderly persons. *Journal of Applied Gerontology* 15:262–76.

Paffenbarger, R. S., Jr., J. B. Kampert, I. M. Lee, R. T. Hyde, R. W. Leung, and A. L. Wing. 1994. Changes in physical activity and other lifeway patterns influencing longevity. *Medical Science in Sports and Exercise* 26:857–65.

Poon, L. W., G. M. Clayton, P. Martin, M. A. Johnson, B. C. Courtenay, A. L. Sweaney, et al. 1992. The Georgia Centenarian Study. *International Journal of Aging and Human Development* 34 (1);1–17.

Poon, L. W., M. A. Johnson, A. Davey, D. V. Dawson, I. C. Siegler, and P. Martin. 2000. Psycho-social predictors of survival among centenarians. In *Centenarians: Autonomy versus Dependence in the Oldest Old,* ed. P. Martin, C. Rott, B. Hagberg, and K. Morgan. Pp. 77–89. New York: Springer.

Williams, L. A., M. A. Johnson, L. W. Poon, and P. Martin. 1995. Oral health and demographic risk factors for poor nutrient intake in the elderly. *Age and Nutrition* 6:4–9.

Yesavage, J. A., T. L. Brink, T. L. Rose, O. Lum, V. Huang, M. Adey, and V. O. Leirer. 1983. Development and validation of a geriatric depression screening scale: A preliminary report. *Journal of Psychiatric Research* 17:37–49.

CHAPTER 10

A Developmental Perspective on Aging and Genetic Technology

A Response to Studies of Centenarians

DIANE SCOTT-JONES, PH.D.

The number of older Americans who reach centenarian status is growing. The Georgia Centenarian Study (Poon et al., 1992) is one of several studies of centenarians, including the New England Centenarian Study (Perls et al., 2002) and studies conducted throughout the world—in Japan (Shimizu et al., 2001, 2002; Willcox, Willcox, and Suzuki, 2001), Italy (Motta, Maugeri, and Malaguarnera, 2002), Sweden (Samuelsson et al., 1997), and Germany Kliegel, Moor, and Rott, 2004). Other studies of older persons include some centenarians, although the 100-year mark is not the exclusive focus; examples are a study of aging nuns (Snowdon, 2003) and the National Survey of Black Americans (Jackson, Chatters, and Taylor, 1993).

At the same time as the number of older persons and their proportion of the population are increasing, genetic technology is advancing and creating both scientific and ethical questions about the new discoveries. Genetic technology might offer prospects for longer, healthier lives. Genetic technology might lead to the eradication of chronic diseases that afflict centenarians as well as those who do not reach centenarian status. The new tools of technology, however, lead to difficult ethical and practical problems that warrant widespread discussion.

Poon's contribution to this volume (chap. 9) asks what we can learn from centenarians, and he offers provocative answers from the Georgia Centenarian Study. Perls (chap. 8) further describes genetic variants and environmental influences that contribute to exceptional longevity. The following commentary focuses on four areas that are of great interest in the study of human development over the lifespan: our understanding of the genetic and environmental components of the correlates of centenarian status; "race" or ethnicity and centenarian status; variability in the developmental pathways to centenarian status; and society's incorporation and accommodation of centenarians.

Genes and Environment

How do new knowledge about genes and new genetic technologies advance our understanding of aging and centenarian status? To answer this question, we can turn our attention to Poon's five predictors of longevity. Three of the predictors of longevity after the first 100 years are social support, nourishment, and cognitive skills. Poon describes these three predictors as "environmentally based." Poon suggests that the remaining two predictors, gender and family longevity, are "genetically based." All five of these predictors, however, can be said to have both genetic and environmental components. These five predictors cannot be divided easily into genetic or environmental camps.

Despite having separated the five correlates of longevity into genetically based or environmentally based categories, Poon emphasizes that heredity, environment, and their interaction contribute to longevity, and he notes briefly the possible biological and genetic contributions to both the length of life and the quality of life. Perls discusses the importance of public health improvements and the promises of mapping longevity-enabling genes. Both authors acknowledge the importance of the *interaction* of biological or genetic contributions with environmental and individual factors in longevity. The strong interactionist view has been discussed by Lewontin (1992), who challenges the notion of genes as causes of disease or disorders. Lewontin points out that a "cancer gene" may have been caused by a person ingesting a pollutant, which may have been caused by an industrial process. Clearly, the ongoing and changing environment contributes to the role of genes in disease and in normal aging.

Heredity and environment are intertwined throughout development. Heredity and environment cannot be usefully separated for complex characteristics that are important in development. Heritability estimates can be misleading. These estimates are sample dependent and refer to percentage of variance in the distribution of a set of scores. Heritability estimates can never allow us to state that, within an individual, a given percentage of longevity (e.g., 30%) is due to heredity and the rest to environment. Nevertheless, Poon suggests that heredity contributes 30 percent and that 70 percent of longevity is "environmentally based." Ultimately, Poon's recommendations are positive and address aspects of the lives of elderly people over which individuals and society can exert some control. Other researchers, in their analysis of the contributions to longevity, also emphasize aspects of elderly persons' lives that are modifiable. For example, Willcox, Willcox, and Suzuki (2001), although they describe biological processes related to centenarians' health, emphasize the modifiable aspects of healthy aging, such as nutrition and exercise, in their 25-year study of longevity in Okinawa. Poon's framing of his recommendations as a partitioning of heredity and environment does not, however, advance our understanding of the role of genes and environment in development (see Lewontin, 1992). Heritability estimates do not answer a developmental question.

The biologist R. C. Lewontin (1992) offers interesting observations on events related to increased longevity. Early in the nineteenth century, deaths in infancy and early childhood reduced the average life expectancy of the overall population. Before the turn of the last century, women had a shorter lifespan than did men; the gender differences reversed, however, when deaths from tuberculosis declined and when young girls no longer experienced burns and scalds from working around open kitchen fires. Lewontin concludes that improvement in nutrition, which is related to increases in income for the masses of people, is associated with increased longevity. He notes that men in the nineteenth century typically were better nourished than women because meat was served to men if the family could afford meat at all. Lewontin further distinguishes between agents and causes. He asserts that underlying social relations in society are causes of health problems that limit survival throughout the lifespan.

"Race"/Ethnicity and Centenarian Status

Studies of centenarians should include careful descriptions of persons who reach this status. Ethnicity or "race" is an important but difficult area to address. Researchers face a conceptual problem in using "race" along with genetic and biological variables in the study of centenarians. "Race" is socially defined but is often used as a biological construct. "Race" has been used in a politicized manner throughout the history of psychology. Common applications of the concept of "race" may suggest that social aspects of development have a biological or genetic basis. Thus, researchers should take care to acknowledge the social use of "race" in studies that address biological and genetic aspects of aging.

In some instances, ancestry and not "race" per se might be more accurate and more relevant in understanding so-called racial or ethnic differences. For example, two centenarian sisters, Elizabeth and Sarah Delany, who wrote two books about their lives, with the assistance of a journalist (Delany, Delany, and Hearth, 1993, 1994), claimed ancestry that included Caucasians and Native Americans as well as African Americans. In a centenarian study, however, these sisters would likely have been classified as African American. Our imprecise and political construction of "racial" categories impedes the scientific study of human development in the latter years as well as in the earlier parts of the lifespan.

Poon found that African-American centenarians had greater depression and poorer self-perceived health than did their Caucasian counterparts. With controls for education and income, however, the difference in self-perceived health disappeared, and the difference in depression diminished but remained significant. Poon does not indicate whether the African-American centenarians with poorer self-perceived health actually had poor health; recall that all centenarians who were studied in the sample were in relatively good health. Further, no clinical depression was found among the Georgia centenarians; therefore, depression could not have been at clinical levels for the African-American participants. Poon does not offer information about gender in this comparison, perhaps because the subsamples of African-American males and females were small. The Georgia centenarians from that particular analysis were predominantly Caucasian, and the "racial" or ethnic comparisons should be interpreted cautiously.

It is noteworthy that the differences between African Americans and

Caucasians diminished or disappeared when controls for education and income were included in analyses. Because of the confounding of "race" or ethnicity and socioeconomic status in our society, findings attributed to "race" or ethnicity typically have a strong socioeconomic component. The important role of education and income in these findings raises the question of why "race" or ethnicity, and not socioeconomic status, is highlighted in the presentation of findings.

To return to the Delany sisters (Delany, Delany, and Hearth, 1993, 1994), these centenarians' autobiographies provide information, although anecdotal, on the experiences of highly educated African-American female centenarians and on centenarians generally. A dentist and a schoolteacher in their working years, the Delany sisters were 103 and 105 years of age when they published their second book. The Delaney sisters' self-perceptions as centenarians were instructive: "No matter how old you get, you think of yourself as young" (Delany, Delany, and Hearth, 1994, 40). Centenarians may think of themselves as they were at earlier parts of the lifespan. Critical components of these centenarians' sense of self may have been forged in earlier years. (See Sneed and Whitbourne, 2005, for models of the aging self.) Older adults tend to maintain a positive sense of self, despite negative stereotypes of older adults and despite the normative physical changes that occur with age (Sneed and Whitbourne, 2005). Others' perceptions of centenarians in general, and of these highly educated African-American female centenarians in particular, may stand in marked contrast to their self-perceptions. Research that focuses on "race" or ethnicity and genetic and biological aspects of aging should be integrated with the careful study of the self perceptions and social contexts of aging persons (see Jackson, 1980, 1988; Jackson, Chatters, and Taylor, 1993).

Variability in Developmental Pathways to Centenarian Status

A major contribution of Poon's chapter is the emphasis on the variability among centenarians. A common misperception regarding the study of genetic and environmental influences is that increased knowledge of these influences will lead to clear prescriptions for a long life. The public may want to know a formula, whether genetic, environmental, or interactionist, for longevity. Poon's work, however, has not led him to a deterministic perspective on longevity. On the contrary, Poon reminds us that many developmental paths lead to centenarian status. In addition to identifying the major factors that predict longevity, research must document the variation that exists among older adults in the pathways that brought them to centenarian status.

The major outcome in Poon's centenarian study is longevity as measured by reaching 100 years of age or by the additional longevity of centenarians after they reach 100 years of age. In addition to 100 years as chronological age, other important outcomes are morale and life satisfaction at 100 years of age. The same developmental principle would apply to these outcomes as well. Many paths can lead to the quality of life we hope would accompany longevity.

Poon raises an intriguing form of the question of variability. Some factors related to centenarian status are also good practices at earlier points in the lifespan. Why, then, do persons who engage in healthful practices not necessarily live to centenarian status? Why do some persons with negative health practices live longer than average? Poon notes that for some centenarians, specific factors may stand out that we would accept as plausible precursors of living to be 100 years of age. Other centenarians, in contrast, may be lifelong smokers and outlive some who do not smoke. For still others, there are no discernible characteristics or behaviors that we would expect to be associated with longevity in a positive or negative direction. As Poon suggests, he may have unraveled some ingredients of longevity, but we are far from a recipe for a long life. This mystery of longevity is part of the complexity of human development over the lifespan. More studies are needed of the multiple pathways leading to centenarian status.

Gender differences may be an important part of the biological and genetic puzzle of longevity, although observed gender differences, of course, have an unavoidable confounding of heredity and environment. Gender differences in reaching 100 years of age are striking. Three-fourths of Poon's centenarians are female.

Region of the country may be a source of variability in the study of centenarians. Poon's centenarian study was conducted in Georgia. Whether the centenarians were born and reared in Georgia, whether they lived in rural areas or urban centers, and other similar variables are important aspects of the variation in centenarians' lives that should be carefully described.

Poon's centenarian study compares independently living (community-dwelling), cognitively functioning 100-year-old persons with two younger groups of persons 80–89 years of age and 60–69 years of age. Knowledge based on only centenarians who are relatively healthy might be misleading. Choosing only centenarians who have no major cognitive impairment and are able to live independently may be a practical and necessary research strategy; however, these selection criteria render meaningless the statements regarding the remarkable good health of the participants. Centenarians in poor health would not have met the inclusion criteria the researchers chose. Poon acknowledges that the findings may not generalize and has a study underway to determine whether findings for "independently living" and "cognitively intact" centenarians generalize to all persons within the age range.

The comparisons of centenarians with persons in their eighties and sixties span four decades. Poon acknowledges the potential cohort effects in these comparisons. Poon reports that centenarians differed from the two younger cohorts on six variables: health and health habits (less smoking, less obesity, less chronic disease, less alcohol, more activity); diet (more carotenoids, vitamin A, whole milk, cholesterol, regular breakfast, and less weight fluctuation); cognition and intelligence (poorer performance except on everyday problem-solving tasks, though education lessened the differences); personality and coping (more dominant, suspicious, practical, relaxed; more acknowledgment of problems and less seeking of social support; more cognitive coping and less behavioral coping); social support (fewer potential visitors but no difference in daily visitors; less likely to talk on telephone or to have spouse as primary caregiver; more likely to have children as caregivers and to receive help with meals from family and friends); mental health (more somatic but not more emotional symptoms). Any or all of these six sets of variables could show cohort effects in addition to providing evidence of correlates of centenarian status.

Dominance and suspiciousness were identified as personality characteristics of centenarians. These characteristics must be assessed carefully, especially in elderly people. Suspicion and dominance may be appropriate in some of the situations centenarians face. Research should assess whether the suspicion and dominance are inappropriate or pathological. The inclusion criteria that limited the centenarian study to relatively healthy persons would suggest that suspicion and dominance were not pathological.

In addition to the cross-sectional comparisons of centenarians with the persons 80–89 years and 60–69 years of age, Poon reports findings of survival analyses. He assessed correlates of the number of days lived after the centenarians reached 100 years of age. Women lived, on average, 34 months after they attained 100 years of age. Men, in contrast, lived an average of 26 months. The gender difference in survival was not significant at 102 years of age but was significant at 103 years. The variables associated with survival past 100 years were social support, sufficient nourishment, and cognition (problem solving, learning and memory, WAIS picture arrangement and block design), which Poon describes as "environmentally based," and gender and family longevity (father's but not mother's age of death), which Poon claims are "genetically based."

To understand the variability of centenarians' experience, we need longitudinal research. The needed longitudinal study, starting at 50 years of age or younger, would be too large and cost-prohibitive and would extend beyond the researcher's career. We need methodologies that include more deep description, case studies of centenarians and those who are approaching the 100-year milestone, and perhaps even systematic study of biographies and autobiographies of centenarians. For example, Coles's (1997) descriptions of men and women over 75 years of age illustrate both the intra-individual and interindividual variability among those approaching centenarian status. We need person-centered methods to supplement the methodologies that rely on identifying a small set of variables associated with longevity.

Society's Accommodation of Centenarians

If more Americans live to 100 years, how will our society incorporate them, and what will be the societal risks and benefits of a higher number and percentage of centenarians? Poon notes that the increase in centenarians has health care, caregiving, economic, social, family, and interpersonal implications.

Findings for centenarians are similar to those from longitudinal studies of health and mortality. Health and longevity are lifelong considerations, not merely concerns that arise in late adulthood. The important aspects of a centenarian's early and midlife are also important throughout the lifespan. Consider, however, the manner in which diet or nourishment played a role in older adults' lives. Currently, for most of the lifespan in our society, from childhood through adulthood, overeating is a severe and wide-

spread problem. Overeating and obesity are associated with life-threatening diseases. The National Center for Health Statistics (2005) found that
40 percent of 55- to 64-year-old Americans were obese in 2003, and 50
percent in that age group have high blood pressure. Although deaths from
heart disease, cancer, and stroke have declined, obesity and other problems, combined with a steadily increasing average lifespan, may mean
that many elderly persons survive with a poor quality of life.

For those who survive to centenarian status, the role of diet changes.
The difficulty becomes undernourishment and not the overnourishment
that now plagues children, adolescents, and adults in the United States.
Eating too much at earlier points in the life course is associated with disease and death. Not eating enough appears to be the problem for centenarians. The number of days of survival past 100 years was positively related
to body fat, body mass, and waist-to-hip ratio. To interpret this finding
fully and to place it in the context of widespread obesity among Americans, more information about the range of body size and the causes of
undernourishment among the elderly is needed.

Centenarians have lived twice as long as the life expectancy for their
birth cohorts. Poon makes the important point that centenarians have lived
through a remarkable range of social and technological change. He notes
that an understudied area is the impact of these lifelong experiences and
critical events on centenarians. We have little research or discussion on
the role of these experiences on current functioning. Centenarians have a
huge accumulation of experiences; they have witnessed many key historical events and great social change.

One set of technological changes that has provided an important context for human development during centenarians' lifetimes is computer
technology. Computer technology has provided a wide range of possibilities for those who live to be 100, but the technology has allowed problems
to flourish as well. For example, electronic mail might allow centenarians
to maintain the social support that is associated with longevity. Older
adults could exchange information and photographs with relatives and
friends, including those who do not live in close proximity. Conversely,
computer technology could be used to accomplish identity theft of centenarians. Centenarians' perceptions of and use of computer technologies is
an important area for study.

Our remarkable advances in computer technology are matched or perhaps surpassed by our strides in human biology and in genetics. Stem cell

research offers many possibilities for enhanced lives for the elderly but also is controversial. Stem cell transplantation has been discussed as a promising therapy for diseases such as Parkinson disease, which affects 2 percent of persons over 70 years of age (National Bioethics Advisory Commission, 1999). Parkinson's is a degenerative brain disease that becomes more difficult to treat as it progresses. If stem cells could be differentiated into brain cells, new brain cells could be created that could be implanted to restore normal function. Beyond the ethical considerations in the creation of stem cells, the cost and availability of new stem cell treatments would be an issue for centenarians.

The possibilities of genetic technologies are extraordinary, and many persons are enamored of high technology. The new frontiers of technology should not cause us to lose sight of other social problems that accompany advancing age and the interests and needs of all age groups in our society. Centenarians were not envisioned when some of our longstanding laws and policies were put in place. As the lifespan increases, laws and policies that were established long ago may need to be revisited to accommodate the increased lifespan.

Increased health care costs have implications for society's support of centenarians and the elderly generally. If health care resources are limited, how will policy makers decide on the allocation of resources to centenarians or to other age groups such as infants? What role will dimensions other than age, such as wealth, play in health care resources for centenarians?

The increase in numbers and percentages of centenarians may strain the social programs that provide for the well-being of elderly persons. In the five-year period from 1997 to 2003, the number of Social Security recipients 85 years of age or older increased at a greater rate than did the number of beneficiaries 65 years of age or older. The rate of increase was 10 percent for recipients 85 years of age and older, in contrast to a 4 percent rate of increase for recipients 65 years of age and older. More than 40,000 centenarians received Social Security benefits in 2002 (Social Security Administration, 2003).

Other examples of potential problems come from the world of work, where tenure and retirement policies may be inconsistent with the likelihood of centenarian status for those who hold "lifetime" appointments. One example of possible problems with lifetime appointments in an era of increased longevity is the appointment of Supreme Court justices. Policies for lifetime appointments to the Supreme Court were established by the Judiciary Act of 1789 (Supreme Court of the United States, 2004). Life expectancy in the United States remained quite low for the next century after the establishment of the Supreme Court. In 1900, life expectancy was 47 years and has risen dramatically to almost 78 years in 2003 (National Center for Health Statistics, 2005). From 1789 to 1970, persons appointed to the Supreme Court served on average 15 years before retiring (Calabresi and Lindgren, 2005). Since 1970, in contrast, Supreme Court justices have served 26 years on average. The average age of justices at retirement has risen from 68 years before 1970 to 79 years since 1971.

According to Calabresi and Lindgren (2005), aging Supreme Court justices have mental incompetence and physical ailments that prevent them performing well. Calabresi and Lindgren propose a constitutional amendment that would prohibit lifetime appointments for justices and would establish 18-year terms. Gruhl (1997), however, reviewed the impact a limited term would have had on previous justices and their decisions. He concluded that term limits might force the best justices to retire too early. The variability among elderly persons that Poon emphasizes in his chapter may contribute to the difficulty of reaching consensus on effective policies for tenure and retirement.

Social support for aging adults might be increased if, as a society, we promoted greater respect for our aging citizens and worked to diminish the stereotypes of and prejudices against elderly people. Hagestad and Uhlenberg (2005) suggest that the age-segregation of the elderly in our society supports negative stereotypes of the elderly. Over time, three-generational households have declined in number but, simultaneously, children have an increased possibility of contact outside their homes with grandparents and great- grandparents because these older relatives are still living. Institutions outside the family that provide support for the elderly typically are age-segregated. Durable family ties across generations and age-integrated settings might increase meaningful social support for elderly adults. Will society develop more positive views of older adults or will we continue as a youth-oriented culture?

Conclusion

Poon has described central developmental themes in his work on centenarians. The themes discussed in this commentary (i.e., the interaction of heredity and environment throughout development, the implications of "race" and other social status variables, the interindividual variability leading to the same developmental outcomes, and society's incorporation of centenarians along with other generations) are deserving of considerable thought. Studying centenarians helps us understand the 100-year point in the life course and the current and possible roles of genetic technology. Research on centenarians also helps illuminate basic developmental principles that apply across the lifespan. Knowledge about genes must be accompanied by knowledge of environments and the strong interaction of genes and environments throughout development. In addition to caring for and assisting elderly people, we as a society can benefit from the wisdom older adults may have gleaned from witnessing and surviving monumental social and technological change.

REFERENCES

Calabresi, S. G., and J. Lindgren. 2005. Term limits for the Supreme Court: Life tenure reconsidered. April 7. http://ssrn.com/abstract=701121.

Coles, R. 1997. *Old and on Their Own*. New York: W. W. Norton.

Delany, A. E., S. Delany, and A. H. Hearth. 1993. *Having Our Say: The Delany Sisters' First 100 Years*. New York: Kodansha America.

Delany, A. E., S. Delany, and A. H. Hearth. 1994. *The Delany Sisters' Book of Everyday Wisdom*. New York: Kodansha America.

Gruhl, J. 1997. The impact of term limits for Supreme Court justices. *Judicature* 81:66–72.

Hagestad, G. O., and P. Uhlenberg. 2005. The social separation of old and young: A root of ageism. *Journal of Social Issues* 61:343–60.

Jackson, J. S. 1980. *Minorities and Aging*. Belmont, CA: Wadsworth.

Jackson, J. S., ed. 1988. *The Black American Elderly: Research on Physical and Psychosocial Health*. New York: Springer.

Jackson, J. S., L. M. Chatters, and R. J. Taylor, eds. 1993. *Aging in Black America*. Newbury Park, CA: SAGE Publications.

Kliegel, M., C. Moor, and C. Rott. 2004. Cognitive status and development in the oldest old: A longitudinal analysis from the Heidelberg Centenarian Study. *Archives of Gerontology and Geriatrics* 39:143–56.

Lewontin, R. C. 1992. *Biology as Ideology*. New York: HarperCollins.

Motta, M., D. Maugeri, and M. Malaguarnera. 2002. Centenarians in good health conditions. *Archives of Gerontology and Geriatrics* 8:209–17.

National Bioethics Advisory Commission. 1999. *Ethical Issues in Human Stem Cell Research*. Rockville, MD: U.S. Government Printing Office.

National Center for Health Statistics. 2005. *Health, United States, 2005*. Washington, DC: U.S. Government Printing Office.

Perls, T. T., J. Wilmoth, R. Levenson, M. Drinkwater, M. Cohen, H. Bogan, et al. 2002. Life-long sustained mortality advantage of siblings of centenarians. *Proceedings of the National Academy of Sciences of the United States of America* 99:8442–47.

Poon, L. W., G. M. Clayton, P. Martin, M. A. Johnson, B. C. Courtenay, A. L. Sweaney, et al. 1992. The Georgia Centenarian Study. *International Journal of Aging and Human Development* 34 (1):1–17.

Samuelsson, S. M., B. Bauer Alfredson, B. Hagberg, G. Samuelsson, B. Nordbeck, A. Brun, et al. 1997. The Swedish centenarian study: A multidisciplinary study of five consecutive cohorts at the age of 100. *International Journal of Aging and Human Development* 45:223–53.

Shimizu, K., N. Hirose, Y. Arai, Y. Gondo, and Y. Wakida. 2001. Determinants of further survival in centenarians. *Geriatrics and Gerontology International* 1: 14–17.

Sneed, J. R., and S. K. Whitbourne. 2005. Models of the aging self. *Journal of Social Issues* 61:375–88.

Snowdon, D. A. 2003. Healthy aging and dementia: Findings from the Nun Study. *Annals of Internal Medicine* 139:450–54.

Social Security Administration. 2003. *Annual Statistical Supplement, 2003*. Washington, DC: Social Security Administration.

Supreme Court of the United States. 2004. A brief overview of the Supreme Court of the United States. March 31. www.supremecourtus.gov/about/institution.pdf.

Willcox, B. J., D. C. Willcox, and M. Suzuki. 2001. *The Okinawa Project*. New York: Clarkson Potter.

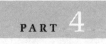

PART 4

GENETIC TESTING

CHAPTER 11

Genetic Testing for Alzheimer Disease

The REVEAL Study

CATHERINE Y. READ, PH.D., R.N.,
J. SCOTT ROBERTS, PH.D.,
ERIN LINNENBRINGER, M.S., C.G.C., AND
ROBERT C. GREEN, M.D., M.P.H.

Alzheimer disease (AD) is a common neurological disorder that accounts for the majority of cases of age-related dementia. It affects more than 4.5 million persons in the United States, and the prevalence of AD is projected to triple by the year 2050 (Hebert et al., 2003). The Alzheimer's Association (www.alz.org) estimates that the annual costs of caring for individuals with AD are at least $100 billion. Researchers in AD are striving to uncover the genetic and environmental correlates of the disease so that effective preventive and treatment strategies may be developed. In this context, identification of specific genotypes that predispose an individual to develop AD may become part of AD risk assessment. As predictive genetic tests become widely available, it will be essential to understand how people respond to risk information, particularly genetic risk information. Clients will need and expect clinicians to help them interpret genetic tests, evaluate risks, and make decisions about health behaviors that could mitigate the onset or course of the disease. In this chapter we will review the neuropathology and natural history of AD, its known genetic and environmental risk factors, and preventive strategies, and discuss the significance of some of the findings of the one of the first studies to examine the impact of genetic risk assessment for AD in asymptomatic persons.

The Natural History of Alzheimer Disease

Dementia is a general term for a syndrome of persistent cognitive impairment in adults. The most common cause of dementia is Alzheimer disease, followed by vascular dementias, Lewy body dementias, frontal lobe dementias, and other etiologies such as depression, tumors, hydrocephalus, and metabolic disorders. The cognitive decline seen in AD is often slow to progress and may at first be difficult to differentiate from normal aging. At present, a definitive diagnosis of AD can be made only at autopsy, when brain tissue is found to contain specific numbers of plaques and tangles. Hence, determining a diagnosis of AD is a clinical process that emphasizes history, physical and mental status examinations, and ancillary diagnostic studies (Green, 2005).

The rate of clinical deterioration in AD progresses slowly at first, then accelerates in the later phases. There do not appear to be pathophysiologic differences between patients with early- and late-onset AD, although persons with the early-onset form may decline at a more rapid rate. For most individuals, AD begins with difficulties in new learning and in the retention of recently learned information. Eventually, deficits in language, visuospatial abilities, or executive functions appear and progress along with worsening memory.

Some individuals exhibit mild cognitive impairment (MCI) before being diagnosed with AD. Individuals with MCI do not meet the criteria for AD or another dementing illness but have a deficit in a particular domain such as memory. Persons with MCI will progress to AD at a rate that is much higher than the incidence rate in the general population, although some persons with MCI do not progress to AD (Petersen, 2004). The classic presentation of early or mild AD involves impaired ability to learn and remember recently learned material, and impairment in at least one other domain such as attention, problem-solving, language, visuospatial function, or praxis. In early AD, which typically lasts one to three years, the individual retains social and conversational skills, and the casual observer may not recognize anything abnormal. As AD progresses to the moderate stage, which lasts two to ten years, deficits in areas other than memory become more obvious. Language and word-finding difficulties exacerbate, and behavioral problems, psychiatric symptoms, and agitation often appear. Simple activities of daily living such as eating, dressing, and walking are impaired by these difficulties and compounded by visuospatial deficits and apraxias. In advanced AD, patients may become incomprehensible or mute. Eventually they deteriorate to a stage of complete helplessness and usually die about eight to ten years after diagnosis, although this is highly variable (Green, 2005).

The Neuropathology of Alzheimer Disease

Tremendous progress has been made in the understanding of the pathologic changes that account for the clinical characteristics of Alzheimer disease (Pasch, 2005). The disorder is characterized by loss of neurons in the cerebral cortex, enlargement of the ventricles, and the presence of neurofibrillary tangles and senile plaques. Tangles are intraneuronal bundles of tau protein, and plaques consist of amyloid-beta (Aβ) peptide core surrounded by neurofibrillary fibers. Aβ is formed when enzymes called secretases break down amyloid precursor protein (APP). Evidence suggests that Aβ accumulation interferes with the synaptic mechanisms necessary for learning and memory, probably by inducing inflammatory changes in brain tissue, damaging neurofibrils, causing the death of neurons, and altering levels of neurotransmitters (Walsh and Selkoe, 2004). Hippocampal function in particular may be compromised by the presence of tangles and plaques; this area of the brain plays an important role in information processing, acquisition of new memories, and retrieval of old memories. AD is associated with a decrease in the activity of choline acetyltransferase, a chemical required for the synthesis of acetylcholine, a neurotransmitter associated with memory, as well as changes in other neurotransmitters.

Risk and Protective Factors for Alzheimer Disease

Certain factors are known or suspected to increase or decrease one's risk of developing AD. Aging is the most dramatic factor associated with increased risk of both dementia and AD. The incidence of dementia doubles every five years between the ages of 65 and 85. A family history of dementia increases the risk of dementia (Green, 2005). Other suspected risk factors include a history of head trauma, female gender, and a history of vascular disease. Possible protective factors include having more years of education, engaging in mentally stimulating activities, and taking anti-inflammatory medications, although the studies supporting these claims must be interpreted with caution (Gatz, 2005).

Genetic Factors

For decades after Alois Alzheimer described the dementing illness that now bears his name, AD was thought to be a rare, noninherited cause of presenile dementia. More recently, studies of families with multiple affected individuals or early-onset AD have informed our understanding of genetic factors that increase disease risk and have led to the current consensus that AD is a common disease with important genetic components (Bird, 2005).

A small number of families exhibit an early-onset form of AD that is transmitted in an autosomal dominant fashion. Mutations in one of three genes (APP, PS1, and PS2) are associated with this rare familial form of AD, in which symptoms typically begin around age 40 or 50. These mutations are referred to as *deterministic,* because their presence guarantees that the affected individual will develop the disease if he or she lives long enough. Genetic testing is available to family members for many of these rare mutations, although its use as a diagnostic or predictive tool remains controversial (Van der Cammen et al., 2004). Preliminary evidence suggests that genetic testing for deterministic AD can be safely conducted (Steinbart et al., 2001).

There is also strong evidence of genetic influence on the development of typical late-onset AD in that family history is a powerful risk factor (Lautenschlager et al., 1996; Green et al., 2002). The most well established polymorphism associated with increased risk of late-onset AD is the apolipoprotein E (APOE) gene on chromosome 19. APOE is a plasma protein synthesized by the liver and also produced by certain brain cells. APOE is involved in the transport of cholesterol and lipids between cells, and is thought to be involved in the pathophysiology of AD through its role in the production of amyloid and the binding of tau. The APOE gene has three co-dominant alleles, e2, e3, and e4, which differ by a single-base substitution in the coding region of the gene. Because each person carries two copies of the APOE gene, there are six possible combinations of the three alleles. The e4 allele has a frequency of about 14 percent in the United States, and its presence increases the risk that an individual will develop AD. In comparison with persons without an e4 allele, someone in his or her sixties with one e4 allele has roughly triple the risk of developing AD, and that risk increases to roughly 15 times in persons with two copies of the e4 allele (Farrer et al., 1997). Despite this increased risk, the presence of the e4 allele does not inevitably lead to the development of AD; even persons with two copies of the e4 allele can live well into their eighties without developing the disease. Thus, the e4 allele of APOE is referred to as a *susceptibility* polymorphism.

The presence of the e4 variant of APOE is an important risk factor for AD, but the fact that it is neither necessary nor sufficient for the development of the disease has fueled the search for other susceptibility genes. Many other genes have been implicated, although sufficient replication has yet to confirm those associations. Because genetic markers associated with increased susceptibility to developing AD may become part of the repertoire of medicine, it will be necessary to understand the best ways to use these tests before they become commercially available.

Prevention and Treatment Strategies

Although genes certainly play an important role in the development of AD, it is now clear that, like virtually every disease, AD has both genetic and environmental components. The challenge is to identify and understand the interactions between those genetic and environmental factors (Bird, 2005). At least for the near future, prevention and treatment efforts will focus on manipulation of environmental rather than genetic risk factors for AD.

For patients who have already been diagnosed with AD, medications that mitigate specific neurotransmitter deficiencies may be prescribed. Cholinesterase inhibitors (donepezil, rivastigmine, and galantamine) and neurotransmitter receptor modulators (memantine) can benefit some patients for a limited period of time, although these effects are modest. Current research is focusing on a number of disease-modifying treatments, particularly ways to reduce the amount of Aβ aggregation in the brain (Christensen and Green, 2005). A number of researchers are striving to discover therapies that would prevent AD or delay its onset. Although no definitive strategies have been developed, there is some evidence that manipulation of specific environmental factors may delay the onset of AD (Mattson, 2004). Dietary modifications proposed to slow progression or reduce the risk for AD include reducing body mass index, restricting calories, ingesting antioxidants such as vitamin E, and supplementing folic acid. In addition to the Aβ modifiers mentioned above, a number of pharmaceuticals are under study for treating or preventing AD, such as statins, anti-inflammatory medications, and others. The Alzheimer's Association (www.alz.org) initiated a "Maintain your Brain" consumer education campaign that recommends mental activity, social involvement, physical activity, and a low-fat, low-cholesterol diet with antioxidant foods and supplements. The National Institute on Aging also released a publication entitled "Can Alzheimer's Be Prevented?" to help educate the public about possible risk reduction strategies.

Interventions that can delay the onset or slow the progression of AD will be of particular importance to those individuals known to be at increased risk. This creates the need for more precise assessments of AD risk to determine who might rationally benefit from such treatments. Genetic testing could help identify "at risk" healthy individuals who are young enough to benefit from an intervention, but the use of such tests has ethical, legal, social, and clinical implications.

Genetic Testing: Concepts and Dilemmas

Genetic tests can be broadly divided into two categories: diagnostic and presymptomatic, and presymptomatic testing may include testing for both deterministic and susceptibility genes. An example of a diagnostic genetic test is the detection of a particular mutation in the CFTR gene on chromosome 7 to confirm the diagnosis of cystic fibrosis in an infant with respiratory disease. Presymptomatic genetic tests, including both deterministic and susceptibility tests, are *predictive* of future disease development, but with different degrees of certainty. An example of a deterministic predictive genetic test would be the detection of the mutation for Huntington disease, because individuals with this gene will ultimately develop the disease if they live long enough. The detection of a susceptibility gene, such as BrCA1 and APOE e4, confers a higher than average risk for breast/ ovarian cancer in the case of BRCA and AD in the case of APOE. Susceptibly genetic testing gives probabilistic information about the risk of developing the disease.

Prediction of risk for adult-onset diseases is by no means a new phenomenon in medicine, but it has historically been based on evaluation of the patient's family history, health practices, signs and symptoms, and phenotypic information obtained though physical examination or diagnostic tests. For example, a positive family history, a history of smoking, and high cholesterol may predict the development of cardiovascular disease. The current revolution in genetics is expanding our ability to predict the occurrence of diseases that have a genetic basis through genotype identification. Genetic information may carry an almost mythical connotation of determinism and has implications not only for the individual patient but also for his or her biologically related family members. Furthermore, there may be a long time delay between the testing and the clinical manifestations of the disease, and there may not be any treatments or modifiable behaviors to mitigate the development of the disease. Finally, unlike other laboratory data, a genetic test can be difficult for medical professionals to understand and communicate owing to its probabilistic nature.

Concerns over the ethical and psychological dangers of genetic testing include the possibility of psychological distress, family discord, inadvertent transfer of risk information to other family members who do not wish to know it, social stigmatization, and insurance or employment bias (Green, 2002). Nevertheless, despite these dangers, there appears to be an acceleration of progress in the identification of both deterministic and susceptibility genes. Concurrently, investment by industry in patenting and marketing as well as popular interest in such tests are increasing at an unprecedented rate.

Debate over the use of genetic tests is intensified by the recognition that recipients of risk information may respond with controversial actions such as suicide or prenatal testing and subsequent termination of pregnancy. Consideration of genetic testing is further complicated by disagreement among health care professionals, as well as the general population, over the value of disclosing risk information to otherwise healthy individuals, particularly in the absence of interventions proven to prevent or delay the clinical onset and/or improve the prognosis of the condition in question (Burke, Pinsky, and Press, 2001). The fact that genetic testing can offer risk information years or even decades in advance of the appearance of recognizable symptoms, particularly in degenerative or later-onset chronic diseases, not only makes accurate validation of these tests difficult but also challenges the wisdom of saddling asymptomatic individuals with many years of possibly inaccurate expectation.

The debate is particularly heated when the risk information is based on

susceptibility genes rather than deterministic genes. Genotyping to identify susceptibility genes provides estimations of risk that are, by definition,
influenced by other genes and nongenetic environmental exposures. This
type of information, though technically "genetic," does not carry nearly
the same degree of certainty as genotyping deterministic genes, where the
presence (or absence) of specific mutations can be unequivocally associated with the future manifestation (or not) of a specific disease. Moreover,
susceptibility genes are likely to be far more common than deterministic
genes, particularly in the late-onset diseases. Thus, susceptibility genotyping is much closer to the kind of information already available to patients
on the basis of family history, environmental exposures, and health-related
behaviors (i.e., a probabilistic estimate of future disease). Studies of patients
and families with other genetic diseases provide insight into the issues
that arise when asymptomatic individuals obtain risk assessment on the
basis of genetic testing.

Lessons from Other Adult-Onset Genetic Disorders: Huntington Disease and Cancer

Huntington disease (HD) is the one late-life disorder in which protocols for presymptomatic, predictive testing have been extensively applied.
Highly accurate predictions for at-risk family members of HD patients was
made possible by the identification of the specific gene responsible for the
disease. A review of the literature about genetic testing for HD revealed
the following: (1) although initial interest in having the test is high, uptake
rates are relatively low (9–20%); (2) people who choose to pursue testing
generally show better psychological functioning than at-risk persons who
decline testing; (3) people receiving results via linkage analysis (less certainty in the test) show better psychological outcomes than those receiving results through mutation detection (more certainty in the test); (4) carriers experience greater transient distress in the weeks following disclosure
of risk, but by six months both carriers and noncarriers are similar and
generally without significant negative psychological effects of testing; and
(5) psychological adjustment at baseline (e.g., level of depression or hopelessness) is a better predictor of post-test adjustment than the test result
itself (Meiser and Dunn, 2000). A more recent qualitative study (Taylor,
2004) corroborated these findings and further concluded that participants
evaluated the test options according to their perception that the test held

value to themselves and/or to a significant other, and to the degree to which they could tolerate and manage the genetic information.

While HD is an example of deterministic testing, there is a growing literature assessing both the pre-test perceptions of, and the post-test response to, genetic susceptibility testing. Most disorders for which such testing is available are types of cancer in which specific mutations or polymorphisms have been identified, notably colon, breast, and ovarian cancers. A review of the literature on psychosocial issues associated with genetic testing for breast and ovarian cancer revealed the following: (1) a positive test for a breast cancer mutation may evoke a psychological response similar to the actual diagnosis of breast cancer; (2) even individuals with a negative result may require psychosocial services; and (3) genetic test results, even if only probabilistic, often form the basis of health care decisions. These conclusions highlight the overall importance of future study of the impact of predictive, presymptomatic genetic testing (Pasacreta, 2003).

The Debate about APOE Testing

Several consensus statements (Brodaty et al., 1995; Farrer et al., 1995; Lovestone, 1995 ; Post et al., 1997; Relkin and Gandy, 1996) have recommended against the disclosure of APOE genotype in asymptomatic individuals in view of the predictive imprecision of the test, the lack of prevention or treatment options, the potential for misuse of the information, and the psychosocial consequences such as fear and worry (Burke, 2002). However, most of these statements concluded that additional research is needed on how probabilistic genetic information about APOE and AD risk is interpreted and used.

There are also compelling arguments in favor of APOE testing and disclosure. There is substantial evidence that even in the absence of accepted treatments or prevention options, individuals desire genetic test results for a variety of medical and nonmedical reasons (Roberts, 2000; Roberts et al., 2003). Treatments to modify the risk or delay the onset of Alzheimer disease are under investigation and may become available in the relatively near future (Green, 2002), and APOE disclosure could significantly enrich prevention trials by targeting at-risk individuals. Any therapy that slowed the progression or delayed the onset of AD would significantly reduce the burdens and costs associated with it (Brookmeyer, Gray, and Kawas, 1998), especially if it was possible to target individuals with the greatest risk. A large-scale treatment trial for individuals with MCI suggested a differential short-term response to medication (in this case, donepezil) by APOE genotype (Petersen et al., 2005).

The REVEAL Study

The Risk Evaluation and Education for Alzheimer's Disease (REVEAL) Study is an ongoing, multisite randomized clinical trial designed to evaluate the psychological and behavioral impact of genetic risk assessment with disclosure of APOE. REVEAL has been funded since 1999 by the National Human Genome Research Institute and the National Institute on Aging. In the initial phase, several large-scale epidemiological data sets representing thousands of family members were combined to generate gender and genotype-specific risk curves suitable for disclosure (Cupples et al., 2004). An example of a risk curve for men who are first-degree relatives of patients with AD and who have one e4 allele is shown in figure 11.1. Those with the e3/ e4 genotype have an increased risk after age 55.

In the next phase of the REVEAL Study, a protocol for screening participants and conducting risk assessment and communication was developed and tested. A randomized, controlled trial was then conducted, in which first-degree relatives of patients with AD received genetic risk assessment with or without APOE disclosure. In the Intervention Arm, participants received genetic counseling and risk assessment based on their gender, family history of AD, and APOE genotype. Control Arm participants received genetic counseling and risk assessment based on only their gender and family history. Follow-up for all participants included sessions at six weeks, six months, and one year.

At the start of the REVEAL Study, it was unclear whether anyone would actually be interested in genetic susceptibility testing for AD. Preliminary survey data had indicated that a substantial proportion of first-degree relatives of AD patients reported that they would be interested in pursuing such testing (Roberts, 2000), but the Huntington disease experience showed that far fewer people actually pursued testing than indicated an interest in doing so (Meiser and Dunn, 2000). Because recruitment methods may affect a person's interest in and completion of a research study, a distinction was made between *systematically contacted* and *self-referred* participants.

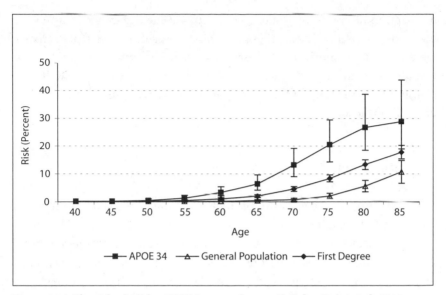

Figure 11.1. The risk of AD by APOE in men. *Source:* Cupples, L. A., et al. 2004. Estimating risk curves for first-degree relatives of patients with Alzheimer's disease: The REVEAL Study. *Genetics in Medicine* 6(4):194. Reprinted with permission, Lippincott, Williams and Wilkins.

To recruit the systematically contacted group, 110 adult children of AD patients were approached who were listed in research registries at each of three sites (Boston University, Cornell University, and Case Western Reserve University). The self-referred group initially consisted of 179 persons who volunteered themselves after learning about our study in clinics, public procontations, or through the media. Both subsamples were predominantly white, college-educated persons with a median annual income of at least $50,000. Compared with the systematically contacted group, the self-referred participants were slightly younger (mean age of 53 years), of higher socioeconomic status, and more likely to be women (79% versus 58%; Roberts et al., 2004).

After the initial screening and education protocols, 47 systematically contacted and 115 self-referred participants continued to randomization into either the Intervention or the Control Arm of the study. Ninety-one percent (N = 147) of all enrolled participants completed the 12-month follow-up. Nearly a quarter of all systematically contacted and 60 percent of self-referred participants proceeded from initial contact through randomization in the study (Roberts et al., 2004). The difference in uptake in the two groups is not surprising, because the self-referred participants were proactively motivated to learn their risk. The uptake among the systematically contacted REVEAL Study participants is similar to a 30 percent uptake in a study of first-degree relatives of patients with hereditary nonpolyposis colorectal cancer (Codori et al., 1999).

Reasons for Seeking Genetic Risk Assessment and Continuing with the Study Protocol

Investigators in the REVEAL Study also explored the stated reasons for seeking genetic testing by asking participants to rate the importance of 12 possible reasons why they might want to seek genetic risk assessment for AD. Commonly endorsed reasons included (1) to arrange personal affairs, (2) the hope that effective treatment will be developed, (3) to arrange long-term care, (4) to prepare my family for the possibility of my illness, (5) to do things sooner than planned, and (6) relief if I learned I was at lower risk. We were also interested in learning what motivated participants to continue in the study once they were enrolled. The strongest predictors of progression through disclosure of APOE status included a desire to prepare the family for AD, a wish to contribute to AD research, the desire to arrange personal affairs and long-term care, and to learn information for future family planning. Hence, at-risk individuals pursue AD susceptibility testing for a variety of (mostly nonmedical) reasons, even in the relative absence of available treatments (Roberts et al., 2003).

The Impact of Receiving APOE Results

Before the REVEAL Study, no data were available on the psychological or behavioral consequences of providing genetic risk assessment for AD with APOE genotyping. The design of the REVEAL Study allowed outcomes to be measured and compared in participants who were randomized to the Intervention Arm (where risk assessment included APOE results) versus those randomized to the Control Arm (where risk assessment was based primarily on family history). Comparisons were also made between participants who received disclosure of a positive test for e4 and those who received a negative test for e4. Among the participants in the Intervention Group in whom APOE genotype was eventually disclosed as part of the risk assessment protocol, 48.6 percent were "e4-positive" because they had either one or two e4 alleles.

The REVEAL Study incorporated several outcome measures that are helping us to understand the overall impact of APOE testing. The psychological impact was evaluated using measures of anxiety, depression, impact of the event, personal assessment of risk, likelihood of participating again, and recall of risk information. The behavioral impact was evaluated using measures of health behavior change and insurance purchasing. Anxiety and depressive affect were evaluated after risk assessment for AD using the Beck Anxiety Inventory (BAI; Beck, Brown, and Steer, 1988) and the Center for Epidemiological Studies Depression Scale (CES-D; Radloff, 1977). The Impact of Event Scale (IES; Horowitz, Wilner, and Alvarez, 1979) is a 15-item self-report measure that assesses two common responses related to a specific stressful life event: intrusion and avoidance.

A comparison of participants in the Intervention Group versus the Control Group revealed no significant difference in change score on the BAI or CES-D at 6 weeks, 6 months, or 12 months. There were also no significant differences in scores between the e4-positive and e4-negative groups. All group means were well below clinical cutoff scores for anxiety and depression at the three time points. This suggests that as a group, those who received genotype disclosure did not experience adverse psychological outcomes as compared with controls, regardless of the outcome of the test (Roberts et al., 2005). The e4-positive individuals scored higher on the IES than their e4-negative counterparts at 6 weeks, 6 months, and 12 months, indicating a higher level of distress; however, all group means were below the cutoff scores considered to be clinically significant (Roberts et al., 2005).

The Effect of Genotype Information on Perception of Risk

Six weeks after risk disclosure, participants were asked to rate their belief that they would develop AD and their postdisclosure changes (if any) in anxiety and personal sense of risk (LaRusse et al., 2005). Data were used from 66 women who had received a 29 percent lifetime risk estimate of developing AD to determine whether responses differed between those who had received a negative e4 result and those who had been given the exact same estimate based on family history. There were significant differences between the two groups on all three items. Thirty-six percent of the family history group believed that they would develop AD, compared with 13 percent of those who had received a negative e4 result. Sixty-seven percent of the negative genotype group reported lower anxiety since getting the test result, compared with 26 percent of those with no test result. Finally, 73 percent of the negative genotype group and 25 percent of the family history group reported a lower personal sense of risk for AD since disclosure. These findings indicate that adding the negative result of a genetic susceptibility test to risk disclosure can decrease the person's estimate of disease risk and decrease the anxiety associated with that perception. Interestingly, this impact was not observed when the participant received a positive genetic test result in comparison with those who did not receive any genetic test result.

Changes in Insurance after APOE Disclosure

Given the concern about the impact of genetic testing for adult-onset diseases on the insurance industry, it was of interest whether participants made changes to their health, life, disability, or long-term insurance following risk assessment for AD. Relatively few participants reported making changes in their health, life, or disability insurance in the 12 months following risk disclosure. However, 17 percent of the e4-positive group (compared with 2 percent of the e4-negative group and 4 percent of the controls) reported making changes in their long-term care insurance. Forty-six percent of the e4-positive group reported "thinking about" making a change in long-term care insurance, compared with 22 percent of the e4-negative group and 33 percent of the controls (Zick et al., 2005). Policy makers may need to address issues of genetic discrimination and adverse selection in insurance markets as susceptibility testing for common, complex diseases is increasingly incorporated into health care.

Conclusion

The REVEAL Study pioneered the use of a real-life susceptibility testing paradigm for Alzheimer disease. The data thus far indicate that genotype information can be disclosed safely and meaningfully if appropriate education and genetic counseling are provided. Participants alter their health behaviors and insurance purchasing practices based on genotype disclosure, and they are satisfied with the risk assessment protocol. These findings provided the groundwork for current and future iterations of REVEAL, which will explore the issues of racial and social identity, the use of alternative protocols, and the long-term impact of genetic risk assessment.

A current focus of the REVEAL Study is to examine perceptions of genetic testing and responses to APOE disclosure among African Americans. Lifetime risk curves have been estimated, and the risk of dementia among first-degree relatives of AD patients is higher among African Americans than among European Americans (Green et al., 2002). African Americans may view the risks and benefits of genetic testing differently from other racial/ethnic groups (Hipps, Roberts, and Green, 2003), a finding that supports the need for investigation of cultural diversity issues with regard to genetic testing.

The REVEAL Study is currently completing a new clinical trial to compare the original education and disclosure protocol with a more clinically feasible "compressed" protocol. The results of this trial will be important information if and when presymptomatic genetic testing for adult-onset diseases becomes part of routine medical practice.

Another important consideration in designing disclosure protocols is that APOE has been linked to cardiovascular risk as well as risk of AD. This characteristic, known as genetic pleiotropy, is a common occurrence, yet there has been little research done on how clinicians might approach the communication of pleiotropic risk with specific genetic markers. APOE affords a unique opportunity to evaluate this question.

A new clinical trial is planned in which all participants receive APOE disclosure but are randomized to receive risk information on AD alone or pleiotropic risk information about AD and cardiovascular disease, using the same outcome measures of anxiety, affect, and other behaviors.

Also of interest is the appropriateness of APOE testing in persons with mild cognitive impairment, a condition that increases the probability of developing AD. It is likely that persons with MCI will be recruited for studies of potential treatments, and APOE disclosure may be included in those protocols. However, there have never been any studies examining the understanding, psychological impact, or subsequent behavior of individuals with MCI who receive genetic risk assessment. The REVEAL Study plans to generate risk estimates that incorporate the presence or absence of MCI as well as age, gender, race, family history, and APOE genotype.

Combining genotype information with probabilistic phenotypic information would more closely approximate the true risk of a disease with both
genetic and environmental correlates.

Finally, there is a need to study the long-term impact of genetic risk
assessment for AD, an adult-onset disease with an unpredictable course
and severity. The REVEAL Study plans to reexamine participants who
were enrolled as early as 2000 to determine whether there are differences
between those who test positive and negative for APOE on scales of anxiety and affect. Long-term studies such as this are essential to our understanding of the real impact of genetic disclosure.

ACKNOWLEDGMENTS

Supported by NIH grants RO1-HG/AG02213 (the REVEAL Study), P30-AG13846
(Boston University Alzheimer's Disease Core Center), and M01-RR00533 (Boston
University General Clinical Research Center).

REFERENCES

Beck, A. T., G. Brown, and R. A. Steer. 1988. An inventory for measuring clinical
anxiety: Psychometric properties. *Journal of Consulting and Clinical Psychology* 56:893–97.

Bird, T. D. 2005. Genetic factors in Alzheimer's disease. *New England Journal of
Medicine* 352:862–64.

Burke, W. 2002. Genetic testing. *New England Journal of Medicine* 347:1867–75.

Burke, W., L. E. Pinsky, and N. A. Press. 2001. Categorizing genetic tests to identify
their ethical, legal, and social implications. *American Journal of Medical Genetics* 106:233- 40.

Brodaty, H., M. Conneally, S. Gauthier, C. Jennings, A. Lennox, and S. Lovestone.
1995. Consensus statement on predictive testing for Alzheimer disease. *Alzheimer Disease and Associated Disorders* 9:182–87.

Brookmeyer, R., S. Gray, and C. Kawas. 1998. Projections of Alzheimer's disease in
the United States and the public health impact of delaying disease onset. *American Journal of Public Health* 9:1337–42.

Christensen, D. D., and R. C. Green. 2005. Disease-modifying therapy for Alzheimer's disease: Update on emerging treatments. *CNS News,* November, 21–26.

Codori, A. M., G. M. Petersen, D. L. Miglioretti, E. K. Larkin, M. T. Bushey, C. Young,
et al. 1999. Attitudes toward colon cancer gene testing: Factors predicting test
uptake. *Cancer Epidemiology, Biomarkers, and Prevention* 8:345–51.

Cupples, L. A., L. A. Farrer, A. D. Sadovnick, N. Relkin, P. Whitehouse, and R. C. Green. 2004. Estimating risk curves for first-degree relatives of patients with Alzheimer's disease: The REVEAL study. *Genetics in Medicine* 6(4): 192–96.

Farrer, L. A., M. F. Brin, L. Elsas, et al. 1995. Statement on use of apolipoprotein E testing for Alzheimer disease. *Journal of the American Medical Association* 274:1627–29.

Farrer, L. A., L. A. Cupples, J. L. Haines, B. Hyman, W. A. Kukull, R. Mayeux, et al. 1997. Effects of age, sex, and ethnicity on the association between apolipoprotein E genotype and Alzheimer's disease: A meta-analysis. *Journal of the American Medical Association* 278:1349–56.

Gatz, M. 2005. Educating the brain to avoid dementia: Can mental exercise prevent Alzheimer disease? *PLoS Medicine* 2(1):38–40.

Green, R. C. 2002. Risk assessment for Alzheimer's disease with genetic susceptibility testing: Has the moment arrived? *Alzheimer's Care Quarterly* 3:208–14.

Green, R. C. 2005. *Diagnosis and Management of Alzheimer's Disease and Other Dementias,* 2nd ed. Caddo, OK: Professional Communications.

Green, R. C., L. A. Cupples, R. Go, K. S. Benke, T. Edeki, P. A. Griffith, et al. 2002. Risk of dementia among white and African American relatives of patients with Alzheimer disease. *Journal of the American Medical Association* 287:329–36.

Hebert, L. E., P. A. Scherr, J. L. Bienias, D. A Bennett, and D. A. Evans. 2003. Alzheimer disease in the US population: Prevalence estimates using the 2000 census. *Archives of Neurology* 60:1119–22.

Hipps, Y. G., J. S. Roberts, and R. C. Green. 2003. Differences between African Americans and whites in their attitudes toward genetic testing for Alzheimer's disease. *Genetic Testing* 7(1):39–44.

Horowitz, M., N. Wilner, and W. Alvarez. 1979. Impact of Event Scale: A measure of subjective stress. *Psychosomatic Medicine* 41(3):209–18.

LaRusse, S., J. S. Roberts, T. M. Marteau, H. Katzen, E. Linnenbringer, M. Barber, et al. 2005. Genetic susceptibility testing versus family history–based risk assessment: Impact on perceived risk of Alzheimer disease. *Genetics in Medicine* 7(1): 40–53.

Lautenschlager, N. T., L. A. Cupples, et al. 1996. Risk of dementia among relatives of Alzheimer's disease patients in the MIRAGE study: What is in store for the oldest old? *Neurology* 46:641–50.

Lovestone, S. 1995. The genetics of Alzheimer's disease: New opportunities and new challenges. *International Journal of Geriatric Psychiatry* 10:1–7.

Mattson, M. P. 2004. Pathways towards and away from Alzheimer's disease. *Nature* 430:631–39.

Meiser, B., and S. Dunn. 2000. Psychological impact of genetic testing for Huntington's disease: An update of the literature. *Journal of Neurology, Neurosurgery, and Psychiatry* 69:574–78.

Pasacreta, J. 2003. Psychosocial issues associated with genetic testing for breast and ovarian cancer risk: An integrative review. *Cancer Investigation* 2:588–623.

Pasch, S. K. 2005. Disorders of thought, mood, and memory. In *Pathophysiology: Concepts of Altered Health States,* 7th ed., ed. C. M. Porth. Pp. 1265–87. Philadelphia: Lippincott, Williams and Wilkins.

Petersen, R. C. 2004. Mild cognitive impairment as a diagnostic entity. *Journal of Internal Medicine* 256:183–94.

Petersen, R. C., R. G. Thomas, M. Grundman, D. Bennett, R. Doody, S. Ferris, et al. 2005. Vitamin E and donepezil for the treatment of mild cognitive impairment. *New England Journal of Medicine* 352:2379–88.

Post, S. G., P. J. Whitehouse, R. H. Binstock, S. K. Eckert, L. A. Farrer, et al. 1997. The clinical introduction of genetic testing for Alzheimer disease: An ethical perspective. *Journal of the American Medical Association* 277:832–36.

Radloff, L. S. 1977. The CES-D Scale: A self report depression scale for research in the general population. *Applied Psychological Measurement* 1:385–401.

Relkin, N. R., and S. Gandy. 1996. Consensus statements on the use of APOE genotyping in Alzheimer's disease. *Neurology Alert* 14:58–59.

Roberts, J. S. 2000. Anticipating response to predictive genetic testing for Alzheimer's disease: A survey of first-degree relatives. *Gerontologist* 40:43–52.

Roberts, J. S., M. Barber, T. Brown, L. A. Cupples, L. A. Farrer, S. LaRusse, et al. 2004. Who seeks genetic susceptibility testing for Alzheimer's disease? Findings from a multisite, randomized clinical trial. *Genetics in Medicine* 6(4):197–203.

Roberts, J. S., L. A. Cupples, N. R. Relkin, P. J. Whitehouse, and R. C. Green. 2005. Genetic risk assessment for adult children of people with Alzheimer's disease: The Risk Evaluation and Education for Alzheimer's Disease (REVEAL) Study. *Journal of Geriatric Psychiatry and Neurology* 18:250–55.

Roberts, J. S., S. LaRusse, H. Katzen, P. J. Whitehouse, M. J. Barber, S. Post, et al. 2003. Reasons for seeking genetic susceptibility testing among first-degree relatives of people with Alzheimer disease. *Alzheimer Disease and Associated Disorders* 17(2):86–93.

Steinbart, E. J., C. O. Smith, P. Poorkaj, and T. D. Bird. 2001. Impact of DNA testing for early-onset familial Alzheimer disease and frontotemporal dementia. *Archives of Neurology* 58:1828–31.

Taylor, S. D. 2004. Predictive genetic test decisions for Huntington's disease: Context, appraisal, and new moral imperatives. *Social Science and Medicine* 58(1): 137–49.

Van-der-Cammen, T. J., E. A. Croes, B. Dermaut, M. C. deJager, M. Cruts, C. Van-Broeckhoven, and C. M. Van-Duijn. 2004. Genetic testing has no place as a routine diagnostic test in sporadic and familial cases of Alzheimer's disease. *Journal of the American Geriatrics Society* 52:2110–13.

Walsh, D. M., and D. J. Selkoe. 2004. Deciphering the molecular basis of memory failure in Alzheimer's disease. *Neuron* 44(1):181–93.

Zick, C. D., C. J. Mathews, J. S. Roberts, R. Cook-Deegan, R. J. Pokorski, and R. C. Green. 2005. Genetic testing for Alzheimer's disease and its impact on insurance purchasing behavior. *Health Affairs* 24:483–90.

CHAPTER 12

The Implications of Genetic Testing for Alzheimer Disease

MARGARET GATZ, PH.D., AND
JESSICA BROMMELHOFF, M.A., M.P.H.

The idea that one might develop dementia tends to be among the more frightening prospects for individuals contemplating their own aging. In particular, having a family member who has dementia can lead to the concern that one is now looking directly into one's own future. Genetic testing offers the promise of giving more individualized information about personal risk. In chapter 11 of this volume Read and colleagues describe the innovative REVEAL Study, in which individuals were randomized such that one group received apolipoprotein E genotype disclosure and counseling while another group received counseling based on family history only. This chapter discusses a number of issues that warrant consideration in planning ahead for a time when genetic testing for dementia risk may become more common.

Alzheimer Disease and Dementia

It is important to distinguish between genetic testing for Alzheimer disease (AD) and genetic testing for dementia. Genetic testing is necessarily specific to one disease or to one type of dementia. The term *dementia* refers to a group of diseases, all of which entail progressive impairment in multiple cognitive areas. Within this group of diseases, AD comprises about two-thirds of all cases of dementia (Geldmacher and Whitehouse, 1996). Thus, results of genetic testing for AD would only partially inform people about their risk of developing dementia. This distinction is important because the question most people ask is not whether they are going to develop AD but rather whether they are at risk of developing dementia. This distinction makes education about the meaning of genetic test results (or the meaning of a positive family history) even more complicated, as it is necessary to inform the individual of the precise meaning of genetic susceptibility as well as the fact that dementia does not always connote AD.

Genetics and Alzheimer Disease

Genetic factors play a large role in the etiology of AD. In what has sometimes been called familial AD, there is a clear pattern of autosomal dominant inheritance and most often an age of onset prior to age 60. However, familial AD accounts for at most only 3 percent of all cases of AD and is related to a point mutation on chromosome 21, 4, or 1, affecting amyloid precursor protein, presenilin 1, or presenilin 2, respectively (Ashford and Mortimer, 2002). For this minority, knowing that one has inherited the deterministic gene variant can lead to a clear expectation that the individual will manifest AD, with onset as early as the fourth or fifth decade of life.

For those with what has sometimes been called sporadic AD, onset tends to be later, and there is no specific gene identified that causes the disease. Among those with sporadic AD, only 25 percent have had a close relative with dementia (Bird, 2005). Nonetheless, it is estimated that at least 50 percent of the explanation is genetic (Ashford and Mortimer, 2002). These genetic influences reflect multiple genes that each influence probability of developing AD. Specific regions of DNA that affect a measured trait (such as AD) are referred to as quantitative trait loci (QTLs). Unlike the definitive gene variants, having one of these genes does not make disease inevitable; rather, it quantitatively alters one's risk.

One basis for estimating the role of genetic influences on a disease is the results of twin studies, where concordance rates for AD between monozygotic (identical) twins tend to be between 60 percent and 80 percent and concordance rates for AD between dizygotic (fraternal) twins are between 25 percent and 30 percent (Bergem, Engedal, and Kringlen, 1997; Gatz et al., 2005). Concordance rates for dementia in twin studies are largely driven by concordance for AD, with very low concordance observed for vascular dementia (Bergem, Engedal, and Kringlen, 1997).

The most apparent genetic factor associated with the heritability of Alzheimer disease is an allele variant, apolipoprotein E (APOE) e4. APOE e4 has been estimated to account for anywhere between 15 percent and 50 percent of sporadic AD in the United States and Europe (Ashford and Mortimer, 2002; Plomin and McGuffin, 2003; Reynolds, Wetherell, and Gatz, 1999). As opposed to the deterministic gene variants that explain familial AD, the APOE e4 allele is a susceptibility marker for AD. Positive testing results do not definitively reveal whether a person will eventually develop AD, and the absence of this gene does not mean a person will not develop dementia (Green, 2002). Furthermore, the APOE e4 allele is not the only gene influencing the risk of sporadic AD. Bird (2005) contends that there may be two to six additional genes that increase the risk of developing AD and have some bearing on the age of onset for the disease; others have suggested that there may be up to 24 additional genes (Ashford and Mortimer, 2002; Rocchi, et al., 2003). As yet, efforts to find other genes have been dogged by inconsistent results and small effects, such as would be expected from QTLs (Plomin and McGuffin, 2003). Genetic susceptibility factors for vascular dementia are largely unexplored, although one would expect that genes related to vascular disease might also affect risk of dementia. Thus, at present APOE is the only susceptibility gene on which genetic counseling about dementia risk could be based. Yet APOE genetic testing results give only incomplete information about genetic risk.

Environmental Factors and Reducing the Risk of Dementia

If 50 percent of the explanation for AD is genetic, then 50 percent is environmental. Once people receive genetic testing results, it seems likely that the next question will be what to do about their risk. Because at present there is no therapy for directly altering the function of APOE e4, the answer to reducing risk of developing AD will necessarily have to focus on environmental factors. We turn now to what is known about environmental risk factors. The etiology of AD is typically portrayed as a composite of genetic and nongenetic factors, although Bird contends that the environmental evidence remains "largely speculative" (2005, 863). Results are often inconsistent, and many factors may be present in so few people as to account for only small proportions of disease risk. However, just as the effects of each gene may be small yet cumulative, the same may be true of environmental factors.

Among the first environmental factors to be studied was head trauma involving loss of consciousness. This is a relatively well established risk factor (Mortimer et al., 1991; Guo et al,. 2000) that may also interact with family history of AD in first-degree relatives (Mortimer, et al., 1998; but see Van Duijn et al., 1994) or with APOE genotype (Mayeux, 2003). Traumatic head injury is an environmental factor about which people can readily take preventive action (e.g., wearing helmets when riding bicycles or motorcycles). However, head trauma accounts for a minor proportion of attributable risk. Mortimer (1995) estimated that the probability of sustaining head injury with loss of consciousness is about 5 percent. Based on the rate of head injury combined with the strength of its association with AD, Mortimer calculated the etiologic fraction, or proportion of cases of AD related to head trauma. He concluded that if head trauma were prevented for all people in the population, only 4 percent of cases of AD would be eliminated (Mortimer, 1995).

Other environmental risk factors are less well established. Attempts to find a viral link have yielded mixed results. For example, the EURODEM Risk Factors Research Group found no relationship between AD and neurotropic virus, meningitis, or encephalitis (Van Duijn and Hofman, 1992). However, there is evidence that herpes simplex virus type I infection may increase the risk of developing AD in people who harbor the APOE e4 allele (Itzhaki et al., 1997; Dobson and Itzhaki, 1999).

Studies of toxins illustrate that despite the absence of consistent results, the general public is quick to embrace a possible means of preventing dementia. In the early to mid–1990s one theory popular in the public domain proposed that consumption of aluminum, for example via drinking water or cooking with aluminum pans, might be a risk factor for cognitive impairment, and in particular AD (McLachlan, Fraser, and Dalton, 1992). Although aluminum in high concentrations is neurotoxic, aluminum as a risk factor for AD has not been consistently substantiated (Graves et al., 1998; Campbell, 2002). Similarly, studies have not established a clear association between dementia and exposure to pesticides (Haan and Wallace, 2004), to industrial or organic solvents, such as aromatic compounds or chlorinated solvents (Kukull et al., 1995; Graves et al., 1998), or to heavy metals, such as iron, lead, or zinc (Haan and Wallace, 2004). Of course, at extreme levels of exposure any of these agents might lead to multiple harmful health effects; however, toxins should be regarded as uncorroborated theories of the prevention of AD.

Low education is a statistically strong and consistent risk factor for both Alzheimer disease and other dementia. Based on surveys of several populations, Mortimer (1995) estimated that low education has high probability of exposure at 70 percent and a mean etiological factor of 0.77, which exceeds that for family history of dementia and head trauma (Mortimer, 1995). Thus, Mortimer estimated that if level of education were increased on a population-wide level, nearly 80 percent of all dementia should theoretically be eliminated.

However, the underlying reasons for the association between low education and dementia remain unclear, and hence also unclear is whether simply increasing level of education would have the suggested preventive effect. The results of studies such as the follow-up of the Scottish Mental Survey of 1932 (Deary et al., 2004) and the Nun Study (Snowden et al., 1996) suggest that differences in cognitive aptitude early in life lead to differences in education and eventually to differences in risk for dementia, and that education is a proxy for those early differences in cognitive aptitude. Deary and colleagues (2004) followed the participants of the Scottish Mental Survey of 1932 to examine how performance on intelligence tests at age 11 related to survival and health at age 80. To look specifically at the relationship between childhood intelligence and risk of dementia, they compared the intelligence scores of individuals who developed late-onset dementia with the scores of those who had not developed dementia. They found that scores on the intelligence tests at age 11 were significantly lower in those who developed late-onset dementia compared with those who did not have dementia at follow-up. Along the same lines, Snowdon and colleagues (1990) compared the linguistic complexity of the autobiographical statements written by 93 nuns on entry into the convent as young adults with their cognitive status approximately 58 years later. They found that low linguistic complexity in early adulthood was a strong predictor for both poor cognitive function and AD later in life. Snowdon and colleagues postulated that the relationship was likely due to cognitive ability early in life, rather than subsequent environmental and lifestyle risk factors experienced later in life, because these women all shared the same environment and lifestyle. Furthermore, the authors suggested that perhaps the sisters with low linguistic ability had lower cognitive reserve, causing them to be more vulnerable to the consequences of the neuropathology that accompanies diseases that lead to dementia.

Risk factors for cardiovascular and cerebrovascular disease have also been implicated as risk factors for dementia. Vascular factors are well-established risks for vascular dementia but until recently were not linked to Alzheimer disease. As suggested by its name, vascular dementia, which accounts for approximately 20 percent of all cases of dementia (Geldmacher and Whitehouse, 1996), entails cerebrovascular disease and would be expected to share risk factors with cardiovascular disease, such as hypertension, high cholesterol, smoking, diabetes mellitus, and a high-fat diet (Roman, 2003). For example, Hebert and colleagues (2000) found that women with hypertension were twice as likely to develop vascular dementia as women without hypertension, and Moroney and colleagues (1999) found that elevated levels of low-density lipoproteins were associated with a higher risk of vascular dementia in older adults.

There is now beginning to be evidence that midlife hypertension is also a risk factor for Alzheimer disease (with blood pressure generally going down prior to actual disease onset) (Launer et al., 2000; Whitmer et al., 2005). A few studies find diabetes to be a risk factor for AD as well as vascular dementia (Xu et al., 2004; Whitmer et al., 2005), although most studies do not (MacKnight et al., 2002; Yamada et al., 2003). Elevated cholesterol and a high-fat diet have been shown to be specific risks for AD in some studies (Czech et al., 1994), but not in others (Tan et al., 2003).

Evidence for Preventive Measures

Based solely on the results of these studies of diverse risk factors, it is difficult to determine where preventive measures should be concentrated. Low education is one attractive target. However, on the one hand, perhaps genetic differences in aptitude underlie both differences in intelligence or linguistic complexity and differences in AD susceptibility, and the association between low education and dementia risk reflects genetic rather than environmental influences. In this case, increasing level of education would presumably be ineffectual. On the other hand, if an environmental intervention is suggested by these findings, it might lie in early childhood education or in even earlier interventions to improve brain development, such as improved maternal and child nutrition (Graves et al., 1996).

Findings that low education is a risk factor for AD have led to an interest in mental stimulation and cognitive exercise as a preventive intervention. The data are summarized in Fratiglioni, Paillard-Borg, and Winblad's (2004) review of epidemiological evidence indicating that those with dementia, including AD, had lower mental and social activity earlier in their lives than those without dementia. There are not as yet, however, clinical trials to support the efficacy of mental exercise as a preventive intervention for dementia (Ball et al., 2002; Fratiglioni, Paillard-Borg, and Winblad 2004; Mohs et al., 1998). Nonetheless, a growing number of trade books, senior citizen classes, and websites imply, some with more caveats than others, that those who follow their cognitive training programs will prevent memory loss and reduce risk of dementia—for example, Gary Small's (2004) *The Memory Prescription;* Lawrence Katz and Manning Rubin's (1999) *Keep Your Brain Alive: 83 Neurobic Exercises;* and the "Use It or Lose It" Mental Exercises for Senior Citizens (n.d.). The extent to which belief in mental exercise has become accepted wisdom, despite the lack of firmer data about efficacy, is illustrated by an editorial in the *Los Angeles Times* that proclaimed, "On the list of medical reassurances as to how we can prevent Alzheimer's disease, working crossword puzzles earns high marks" (Miller, 2005).

A final practical and potentially powerful area for preventive intervention is vascular health. Controlling hypertension may be one of the most important interventions in preventing dementia. Hanon and Forette (2004) report that the randomized placebo-controlled trials Systolic Hypertension in Europe (SYST-EUR) and Perindopril Protection against Recurrent Stroke Study (PROGRESS) provided evidence that antihypertensive medications reduce incidence of dementia. In the SYST-EUR study, Forette et al. (2002) found that calcium channel blocker–based antihypertensive medication, possibly accompanied by an ACE-inhibitor, with or without a diuretic, decreased the incidence of all-cause dementia, including AD, vascular dementia, and mixed dementia, by 55 percent in those who received treatment for an average of four years. Based on these results, they reasoned that if 1,000 patients were treated for five years, 20 cases of dementia would be prevented. Similarly, in PROGRESS, Tzourio and colleagues (2003) found that an ACE-inhibitor-based antihypertensive medication, with or without an accompanying diuretic, reduced risk of dementia by 34 percent and risk of cognitive decline by 45 percent in participants with recurrent stroke and reduced risk of cognitive decline in all participants in the active treatment group by 19 percent.

Whether or not statins used to treat hyperlipidemia reduce the risk of AD remains controversial. There is epidemiological evidence and there are plausible biological pathways, but there is as yet an absence of evidence from randomized clinical trials (Scott and Laake, 2001). Case-control and cross-sectional studies have suggested that statin use may reduce the risk of dementia (Jick et al., 2000; Dufouil et al., 2005) and AD (Wolozin et al., 2000; Green et al., 2006). A three-year prospective study of statin use among the Cache County Study participants, however, did not find any association between the use of statins and subsequent dementia or AD (Zandi et al., 2005).

Communicating Ethically about Environmental Risk

Just as messages about genetic risk need to be crafted carefully and accurately (see Read et al., chap. 11 of this volume), so do messages about the environment—the other half of dementia risk. Here, the kinds of behaviors that predominate in the popular press as ways to prevent dementia may not map well onto the kinds of behaviors that might make the biggest difference in dementia risk. For example, although mental stimulation has garnered much popularity in the public domain as a preventive technique, there is little substantiating clinical evidence for its effectiveness. Furthermore, as Gatz (2005) suggests, encouraging uncorroborated prevention techniques may not only offer false hope but may also cause individuals who do develop dementia to be blamed for their condition, through their failure, for example, to have stimulated their brain enough.

As yet there is no definitive explanation of how environmental factors contribute to dementia risk or how they interact with various genotypes. Controlling vascular risk factors and ensuring proper child and maternal nutrition are measures that could be important in preventing dementia as well as developing and maintaining overall brain health. Because the gene-environment interaction for risk of dementia is not fully understood at this time, these measures need not be enacted solely by those who may have an increased genetic susceptibility for developing dementia.

ACKNOWLEDGMENTS

National Institute of Health Grant R01-AG08724 and T32-AG00037 and Alzheimer's Association Award ZEN-02-3895.

REFERENCES

Ashford, J. W., and J. A. Mortimer. 2002. Non-familial Alzheimer's disease is mainly due to genetic factors. *Journal of Alzheimer's Disease* 4:169–77.

Ball, K., D. B.Berch, K. F. Helmers, J. B. Jobe, M. D. Leveck, M. Marsiske, et al. 2002. Effects of cognitive training interventions with older adults: A randomized controlled trial. *Journal of the American Medical Association* 288:2271–81.

Bergem, A. L., K. Engedal, and E. Kringlen. 1997. The role of heredity in late-onset Alzheimer's disease and vascular dementia: A twin study. *Archives of General Psychiatry* 54:264–70.

Bird, T. D. 2005. Genetic factors in Alzheimer's disease. *New England Journal of Medicine* 352:862–64.

Campbell, A. 2002. The potential role of aluminum in Alzheimer's disease. *Nephrology Dialysis Transplantation* 17(suppl. 2):17–20.

Czech, C., H. Forstl, F. Hentschel, U. Monning, C. Besthorn, and C. Geiger-Kabisch. 1994. Apolipoprotein E–4 gene dose in clinically diagnosed Alzheimer's disease: Prevalence, plasma cholesterol levels, and cerebrovascular change. *European Archives of Psychiatry and Clinical Neuroscience* 243:291–92.

Deary, I. J., M. C. Whiteman, J. M. Starr, L. J. Whalley, and H. C. Fox. 2004. The impact of childhood intelligence on later life: Following up the Scottish Mental Surveys of 1932 and 1947. *Journal of Personality and Social Psychology* 86: 130–47.

Dobson, C. B., and R. F. Itzhaki. 1999. Herpes simplex virus type 1 and Alzheimer's disease. *Neurobiology of Aging* 20:457–65.

Dufouil, C., F. Richard, N. Fievet, J. P. Dartigues, K. Ritchie, C. Tzourio, et al. 2005. APOE genotype, cholesterol level, lipid-lowering treatment, and dementia: The Three-City Study. *Neurology* 64:1531–38.

Forette, F., M. L. Seux, J. A. Staessen, L. Thijs, M. R. Babarskiene, S. Babeanu, et al. 2002. The prevention of dementia with anti-hypertensive treatment: New evidence from the Systolic Hypertension in Europe (SYST-EUR) Study. *Archives of Internal Medicine* 162:2046–52.

Fratiglioni, L., S. Paillard-Bord, and B. Winblad. 2004. An active and socially integrated lifestyle in late life might protect against dementia. *Lancet Neurology* 3: 343–53.

Gatz, M. 2005. Educating the brain to avoid dementia: Can mental exercise prevent Alzheimer's disease? *Public Library of Science Medicine* 2:e7.

Gatz, M., L. Fratiglioni, B. Johansson, S. Berg, J. A. Mortimer, C. A. Reynolds, et al. 2005. Complete ascertainment of dementia in the Swedish twin registry: The HARMONY Study. *Neurobiology of Aging* 26:439–47.

Geldmacher, D. S., and P. J. Whitehouse. 1996. Evaluation of dementia. *New England Journal of Medicine* 335:330–36.

Graves, A. B., J. A. Mortimer, E. B. Larson, A. Wenzlow, J. D. Bowen, and W. C. McCormick. 1996. Head circumference as a measure of cognitive reserve: Association with severity of impairment in Alzheimer's disease. *British Journal of Psychiatry* 1:86–92.

Graves, A. B., D. Rosner, D. Echeverria, J. A. Mortimer, and E. B. Larson. 1998. Occupational exposures to solvents and aluminum and estimated risk of Alzheimer's disease. *Occupational and Environmental Medicine* 55:627–33.

Green, R. C. 2002. Risk assessment for Alzheimer's disease with genetic susceptibility testing: Has the moment arrived? *Alzheimer's Care Quarterly* 3:208–14.

Green, R. C., S. E. McNagny, P. Jayakumar, L. A. Cupples, K. Benke, and L. A. Farrer. 2006. Statin use and the risk of Alzheimer's disease: The MIRAGE Study. *Alzheimer's and Dementia* 2:96–103.

Guo, Z., L. A. Cupples, A. Kurz, S. H. Auerbach, L.Volicer, H. Chui, et al. 2000. Head injury and the risk of Alzheimer disease in the MIRAGE Study. *Neurology* 54:1316–23.

Haan, M. N., and R. Wallace. 2004. Can dementia be prevented? Brain aging in a population-based context. *Annual Review of Public Health* 25:1–24.

Hanon, O., and F. Forette. 2004. Prevention of dementia: Lessons from SYST-EUR and PROGRESS. *Journal of the Neurological Sciences* 226:71–74.

Hebert, R., J. Lindsay, R. Verreault, K. Rockwood, G. Hill, and M. F. Dubois. 2000. Vascular dementia: Incidence and risk factors in the Canadian Study of Health and Aging. *Stroke* 31:1487–93.

Itzhaki, R. F., W. R. Lin, D. Shang, G. K. Wilcock, B. Faragher, and G. A. Jamieson. 1997. Herpes simplex virus type 1 in brain and risk of Alzheimer's disease. *Lancet* 349:241–44.

Jick, H., G. L. Zornberg, S. S. Jick, S. Seshadri, and D. A. Drachman. 2000. Statins and the risk of dementia. *Lancet* 356:1627–31.

Katz, L., and M. Rubin. 1999. *Keep Your Brain Alive: 83 Neurobic Exercises.* New York: Workman.

Kukull, W. A., E. B. Larson, J. D. Bowen, W. C. McCormick, L. Teri, M. L. Pfanschmidt, et al. 1995. Solvent exposure as a risk factor for Alzheimer's disease: A case-control study. *American Journal of Epidemiology* 141:1059–71.

Launer, L. J., G. W. Ross, H. Petrovitch, K. Masaki, D. Foley, L. R. White, et al. 2000. Midlife blood pressure and dementia: The Honolulu-Asia Aging Study. *Neurobiology of Aging* 21:49–55.

MacKnight, C., K. Rockwood, E. Awalt, and I. McDowell. 2002. Diabetes mellitus and the risk of dementia, Alzheimer's disease, and vascular cognitive impairment in the Canadian Study of Health and Aging. *Dementia and Geriatric Cognitive Disorders* 14:77–83.

Mayeux, R. 2003. Epidemiology of neurodegeneration. *Annual Review of Neuro science* 26:81–104.

McLachlan, D. R., P. E. Fraser, and A. J. Dalton. 1992. Aluminum and the pathogenesis of Alzheimer's disease: A summary of evidence. *Ciba Foundation Symposium* 169:87–98.

Miller, K. C. 2005. A 10-letter disease prevented by puzzles. *Los Angeles Times,* March 12, B19.

Mohs, R. C., T. A. Ashman, K. Jantzen, M. Albert, J. Brandt, B. Gordon, et al. 1998. A study of the efficacy of a comprehensive memory enhancement program in health elderly persons. *Psychiatry Research* 77:183–95.

Moroney, J. T., M. X. Tang, L. Berglund, S. Small, C. Merchant, K. Bell, et al. 1999. Low-density lipoprotein cholesterol and the risk of dementia with stroke. *Journal of the American Medical Association* 282:254–60.

Mortimer, J. A. 1995. Prospects for prevention of dementia and associated impairments. In *Promoting Successful and Productive Aging,* ed. L. A. Bond, S. J. Cutler, and A. Grams. Pp. 131–47. Thousand Oaks, CA: SAGE Publications.

Mortimer, J. A., I. Fortier, L. Rajaram, and D. Gauvreau. 1998. Higher education and socioeconomic status in childhood protect individuals at genetic risk of AD from expressing symptoms in late life: The Saguenay-Lac-Saint-Jean Health and Aging Study. *Neurobiology of Aging* 19:S215.

Mortimer, J. A., C. M. Van Duijn, V. Chandra, L. Fratiglioni, A. B.Graves, A. Heyman, et al. 1991. Head trauma as a risk factor for Alzheimer's disease: A collaborative re-analysis of case-control studies. *International Journal of Epidemiology* 20:328–35.

Plomin, R., and P. McGuffin. 2003. Psychopathology in the postgenomic era. *Annual Review of Psychology* 54:205–28.

Reynolds, C. A., J. L.Wetherell, and M. Gatz. 1999. Heritability of Alzheimer's disease. In *Research and Practice in Alzheimer's Disease and Other Dementias,* ed. B. Vellas and L. J. Fitten. Vol. 2, pp. 175–91. New York: Springer.

Rocchi, A., S. Pellegrini, G. Siciliano, and L. Murri. 2003. Causative and susceptibility genes for Alzheimer's disease: A review. *Brain Research Bulletin* 61: 1–24.

Roman, G. C. 2003. Vascular dementia: Distinguishing characteristics, treatment, and prevention. *Journal of the American Geriatrics Society* 51:S296–304.

Scott, H. D., and K. Laake. 2001. Statins for the prevention of Alzheimer's disease. *The Cochrane Database of Systematic Reviews.* www.mrw.interscience.wiley. com/cochrane/clsysrev/articles/CD003160/frame.html.

Small, G. 2004. *The Memory Prescription: Dr. Gary Small's 14-Day Plan to Keep Your Brain and Body Young.* New York: Hyperion.

Snowdon, D. A., S. J. Kemper, J. A. Mortimer, L. H. Greiner, D. R. Wekstein, and W. R. Markesbery. 1996. Linguistic ability in early life and cognitive function and Alzheimer's disease in late life: Findings from the Nun Study. *Journal of the American Medical Association* 275:528–32.

Tan, Z., S. Seshadri, A. Beiser, P. Wilson, D. P. Kiel, M. Tocco, et al. 2003. Plasma total cholesterol level as a risk factor for Alzheimer's disease: The Framingham Study. *Archives of Internal Medicine* 163:1053–57.

Tzourio, C., C. Anderson, N. Chapman, M. Woodward, B. Neal, S. MacMahon, et al. 2003. Effects of blood pressure lowering with perindopril and indapamide therapy on dementia and cognitive decline in patients with cerebrovascular disease. *Archives of Internal Medicine* 163:1069–75.

"Use it or lose it" mental exercises for senior citizens. N.d. www.training-classes. com/course_hierarchy/courses/34__Use_it_ or_Lose_it_Mental_Exercises_for_ Senior_Citizens.php.

Van Duijn, C. M., and A. Hofman. 1992. Risk factors for Alzheimer's disease: The EURODEM collaborative re-analysis of case-control studies. *Neuroepidemiology* 11(suppl. 1):106–13.

Van Duijn, C. M., D. G. Clayton, V. Chandra, L. Fratiglioni, A. B. Graves, A. Heyman, et al. 1994. Interaction between genetic and environmental risk factors for Alzheimer's disease: A reanalysis of case-control studies. *Genetic Epidemiology* 11:539–51.

Whitmer, R. A., S. Sidney, J. Selby, S. C. Johnston, and K. Yaffe. 2005. Midlife cardiovascular risk factors and risk of dementia in late life. *Neurology* 64:277–81.

Wolozin, B., W. Kellman, P. Rousseau, G. G. Celesia, and G. Siegel. 2000. Decreased prevalence of Alzheimer's disease associated with 3-hydroxy–3-methylglutaryl coenzyme A reductase inhibitors. *Archives of Neurology* 57:1439–43.

Xu, W. L., C. X. Qiu, A.Wahlin, B. Winblad, and L. Fratiglioni. 2004. Diabetes mellitus and risk of dementia in the Kungsholmen project: A 6-year follow-up study. *Neurology* 63:1181–86.

Yamada, M., F. Kasagi, H. Sasaki, N. Masunari, Y. Mimori, and G. Suzuki. 2003. Association between dementia and midlife risk factors: The Radiation Effects Research Foundation Adult Health Study. *Journal of the American Geriatrics Society* 51:410–14.

Zandi, P. P., L. Sparks, A. Khachaturian, J. Tschanz, M. Norton, M. Steinberg, et al. 2005. Do statins reduce risk of incident dementia and Alzheimer disease? *Archives of General Psychiatry* 62:217–24.

CHAPTER 13

Genetic Susceptibility to Alzheimer Disease

ANN C. HURLEY, R.N., D.N.SC.
ROSE M. HARVEY, R.N., D.N.SC.
J. SCOTT ROBERTS, PH.D., AND
KATHY J. HORVATH, PH.D., R.N.

Identification of the e4 allele of apolipoprotein E (APOE) on chromosome 19 as the most robust risk factor for developing Alzheimer disease (Pericak-Vance et al., 1997; Roses, 1997) has prompted interest in the use of APOE genotyping in a predictive manner. Clinically, APOE genotyping is currently recommended only as a diagnostic aid in the evaluation of persons with dementia. Indeed, there is consensus among some scientists that APOE genotyping should not be used for predictive purposes in asymptomatic individuals (Brodaty et al., 1995; Farrer, Brin, and Elsas, 1995; Relkin, 1996; Relkin, Kwon, Tsai, and Gandy, 1996; Post et al., 1997), because of possible psychological harm or discrimination in an environment in which no preventative treatments are currently available. These consensus reports by scientists and ethicists were written with the intent to avoid harm but without an empirical basis, because no one had studied the impact of APOE risk disclosure on asymptomatic persons at the time those reports were written.

Research to learn genetic risk for Alzheimer disease (AD) had been limited to survey methods with hypothetical scenarios. Results of an early survey showed interest in seeking AD genetic testing to be high (Green et al., 1997). Another survey positing 100 percent accuracy in test results found that although adults both with and without a parent with AD would consider testing in order to plan for the future, they were concerned about lack of treatment options and the possibility of losing their health insurance (Cutler and Hodgson, 2003). Relatives of persons with AD, however, agreed that the perceived disadvantages of AD genetic testing were largely outweighed by the advantages (i.e., informing later-life decisions and planning for future care; Roberts, 2000).

Lack of empirical data within an actual APOE genetic testing situation and consistent reports from clinicians and researchers that some individuals do wish to learn their own APOE genotype prompted Dr. Robert C. Green of Boston University and his team to study the question of genetic risk assessment. This first NIH-funded randomized clinical trial to explore the impact of APOE disclosure in asymptomatic individuals, the *R*isk *E*valuation and *E*ducation in *A*lzheimer's Disease (REVEAL) Study (Green, 2002), was recently completed (Roberts et al., 2003, 2004, 2005; LaRusse et al., 2005; Marteau, Roberts, LaRusse, and Green, 2005; Zick et al., 2005) and is summarized in chapter 11 of this volume.

The REVEAL Study team included neurologists, psychologists, genetic counselors, ethicists, and legal scholars as well as several of the authors (Farrer, Post, and Relkin) of the major consensus statements that had recommended against APOE disclosure to asymptomatic persons. The REVEAL Study enrolled adult children of persons with AD to (1) learn the characteristics and motivations of persons who chose to obtain risk assessment, (2) determine the psychological consequences of genetic risk assessment, and (3) examine real-life changes in health behaviors and insurance purchases made after learning one's personal risk for AD. The REVEAL Study followed participants for one year and compared outcomes of control participants who were provided with *population-based risk* calculated from family history, gender, and age with intervention participants whose *personalized risk* estimates (Cupples et al., 2004) also included their APOE gene type. Analyses compared participants who learned that they possessed at least one copy of the APOE e4 allele (e4-positive group), those who had no copies of the APOE e4 allele (e4-negative group), and controls who did not receive APOE disclosure. An additional qualitative phase, called the REVEALED (*R*isk *E*valuation and *E*ducation in *A*lzheimer's Disease—Development of an Empirical Model) Project, was partially funded by an Alzheimer's Association grant to Dr. Hurley and superimposed over the ongoing REVEAL Study to better understand the perspectives and beliefs of individual participants by hearing their stories told in semistructured interviews.

In REVEALED (Hurley et al., 2005), we explored qualitatively by interview why people chose to participate in the REVEAL Study and compared those reasons with their motivation obtained quantitatively by survey. In our commentary, we discuss the REVEAL Study in the context of REVEALED data and previously published reports from the REVEAL Study of reasons for seeking genetic susceptibility testing (Roberts et al., 2003, 2004, 2005).

Methods

The REVEALED Project used grounded-theory methods (Glaser and Strauss, 1967; Rempusheski, 1999) to interpret interview data. Grounded-theory methods are derived from social process theory and symbolic interactionism (Blumer, 1969) and were used for this exploration for two reasons. First, a basic tenet of symbolic interactionism is that human beings carry out purposeful actions based on their meanings for the individual (Blumer, 1969). Second, process research, such as grounded theory, has been suggested as a way to examine the dynamic psychoeducational process of genetic counseling (Biesecker and Peters, 2001). Thus, grounded-theory methods were appropriate for studying the process of deciding to participate in AD risk assessment research.

A purposive sample was recruited by REVEAL genetics counselors who identified REVEAL participants likely to agree to share their feelings about being in the study, and then invited them to be interviewed for REVEALED. After obtaining informed consent, a semistructured interview guide was used to elicit information about (1) background, (2) personal experiences, (3) reasons for initial participation and continuation in REVEAL, (4) beliefs about AD causes and risk factors, and (5) genetic knowledge and beliefs regarding AD. Before randomization, REVEAL participants had completed a packet including a 12-item survey in which they responded on a four-point Likert scale by strongly agreeing, agreeing, disagreeing, or strongly disagreeing with proposed reasons why they had sought risk assessment.

TABLE 13.1

Percentage of respondents endorsing reasons for seeking genetic testing for AD

	REVEALED (N = 60)		REVEAL (N = 206)	
	Strongly agree	Strongly disagree	Strongly agree	Strongly disagree
To participate in and contribute to AD research	65.9	0.0	62.1	0.7
To arrange my personal affairs	61.7	1.7	51.5	4.4
The hope that an effective treatment will be developed	60.0	0.0	54.6	2.9
To arrange my long-term care	59.3	3.4	47.1	3.9
To prepare my spouse or children for my illness	48.3	5.2	37.9	7.4
To learn information that may eventually be useful for family planning	45.0	11.7	37.2	15.2
To do things sooner than I had planned to do them in the future	38.3	3.3	34.8	3.9
The relief I would anticipate from learning that my chances are lower than I think	25.4	3.4	27.4	4.4
Curiosity	18.6	15.3	19.5	11.7
The feeling that I am already showing symptoms of the disease	8.3	33.3	6.8	34.5
To confirm the feeling that I am going to get the disease	5.0	43.3	4.9	35.9
To plan for suicide in case I learn my chances are high	3.3	66.7	2.4	78.6

Readers should note that participants responded in the context of a research project rather than an actual clinical interaction. Although the survey data provided some understanding of participants' motivation, we hoped that the qualitative phase of data collection would refine and enrich our understanding of how these decisions for risk assessment were made.

Interviews were recorded and transcribed into a word-processing package. Identifying information was removed, pseudonyms were substituted for names, and the file was converted to a qualitative software package, *The Ethnograph,* to facilitate coding. *The Ethnograph* allowed us to retrieve, organize, and ultimately classify coded segments of text (Miles and Huberman, 1994). A process of basic content analysis of narrative data was carried out. Data were examined for instances of "why" participants enrolled, and codes were assigned. These codes were contrasted across participants and combined into broader, more abstract, descriptive categories (Kearney, 2001) to discover new perspectives from the verbatim accounts in participants' stories. Validity was achieved when two independent reviewers agreed on what was heard while coding the transcripts and by grounding concepts in the respondents' words.

Results

Demographic data were collected immediately after enrollment in the first phase of the REVEAL Study. Of the two recruitment sources, 75 percent were self-referred while 25 percent were systematically ascertained from sites' Alzheimer's Disease Center database and/or Memory Disorder Clinic. Sixty REVEALED participants, representing all three sites (25 in Boston, 20 in Cleveland, and 15 in New York), were interviewed approximately 18 months after completing the motivation survey (Roberts et al., 2003). Demographic characteristics of REVEALED participants were similar to those of the REVEAL sample (N = 206). The sample was middle aged (mean = 54.2, range = 37–76 years), mostly female (86.7%), with advanced education (mean number of years education = 16.9) and a high median household income (greater than $100,000 annually). Most had firsthand knowledge of the clinical progression of AD gained through caring for an afflicted parent (71.7%), 50 percent of whom were living at the time. Half of the participants had more than one relative with a memory disorder.

Quantitative Findings

The 60 REVEALED participants endorsed reasons for seeking genetic susceptibility similar to those of the larger sample (Roberts et al., 2003) in the REVEAL Study (table 13.1). The three most strongly endorsed reasons were (1) to contribute to research, (2) to arrange personal affairs, and (3) to support the hope that an effective treatment would be developed.

Qualitative Findings

We coded 137 stories under the category *Why a participant volunteered for the REVEAL Study.* These codes were classified into increasingly broader descriptive categories and finally into the two constructs, altruism and learning. Learning included the three concepts of planning, prevention, and need to know.

Altruism here means helping others by advancing science. Although altruism did encompass an unselfish regard for others, it often included an element of exchange. Participation was either given in thanks for care provided to the AD afflicted parent or in hopes of receiving benefit, such as information for self and family. Thus, both societal and personal interests, implied or explicitly stated, were embedded in altruism. Being a stakeholder in AD research implied a notion of self-interest, for the participant and/or for future generations, and this notion was intensified because all participants were sons or daughters of persons with AD:

> Gabe stated: "When I came here it was strictly because I realized that I was the prime candidate that might be able to help."
>
> Mary wanted to make a contribution. "I mean it's like you are willing to do anything you can if you feel that you could make a mark or contribution."
>
> Regina specifically wished to help others. "I thought maybe it might help somebody, because we had the two people in our family. But the driving force seemed to be maybe I can help somebody else."
>
> Adele wanted to give back. "I just think that our family would be a great group because they did have the brain autopsy. They did know that was her cause of death and if it was genetic or whatever—that if I could help in anyway I just wanted to return that favor."

Doris hoped that her contribution to science would give meaning to her parent's AD. "I was feeling—and I still feel—like if there's something I can do to try to help advance the knowledge, or the treatment, or the understanding, or some greater good here, if there's any greater good that can come from my father's illness, I'm happy to try to help get to that."

Uri participated for his parent. "For her. Yeah. I think, knowing mom, I mean we knew that she would want to do anything that could help. Which is also why I'm doing this."

Paul was uneasy because of the AD history in his family. "You know, I thought if I can help in any way to do anything to participate in this study, that's all that was important to me. And I said, anything I could do to help. I still feel that way. I have an interest in the disease because my mother has it."

Xylona wanted to help the next generation. "And because my mom had Alzheimer's and I kind of feel that research does help, maybe not in the short-term, but in the long-term. And so maybe it wouldn't be of help for me, but it might be of help for my children or grandchildren, so therefore why not do something that might help somebody else down the line?"

Learning is defined on a continuum from curiosity for self and/or a scientific detached inquisitiveness to a purposive desire to know:

Ora stated succinctly: "Just a desire to know."

Quinsella was interested both personally and scientifically. "Oh, I suppose I've always had the nagging thought in the back of my mind if my mother had dementia of whatever sort, it would be kind of interesting to find out. But also, I'm just plain interested in it from a totally scientific view. I really do love science."

Francine wanted to learn her risk for AD because it may affect how she looks at her life. "I guess I wanted to know, like, what my chances were. And as I said, well, maybe it will make me look at my life in a different way."

Ken also wanted to learn his risk. "You know, I wanted to find out if I was susceptible, you might say, based on genetics. That's why I took the test, to find out."

Anne considered her children. "So I just wanted to know. And usually you can find out the up-to-date type of things they're doing and what they're studying, and stuff like that. I wanted to find out—I wanted to find out what my chances were . . . But I've got two little kids. I want to find out as much as I can."

In addition to talking about wanting to learn, participants talked about why learning was valuable to them. They talked about the need to plan, hope for prevention and just needing to know, perhaps to relieve worries or confirm fears. *Planning* means thinking ahead to consider or make future arrangements for self and while preparing, not burdening others:

> Roberta considered future caregiving needs of herself and her husband. "When they wanted to know if I wanted to do the program I go sure, I want to see where I'm at, you know. Because I can make some decisions in my life that I could take care of everything before and not have everybody else stress about it, you know. So to me, that's when I started. I really feel, hey, my husband was sick, I figured I needed to know because what if I get it? Who's going to take care of me? You know, and then I wasn't worried who was going to take care of me, who's going to take care of him?"

> Henrietta wanted to be prepared. "Because I wanted to know. Because if I have a high risk for Alzheimer's, there are a lot of things that I want to get in order that I might just let slide. There are some things that I haven't done that I may want to start doing, and also to inform my spouse that if he starts seeing signs of this, let me know so I can speed up the schedule, you know, of getting my will done and that sort of thing."

Prevention means reducing one's risk for AD. Prevention was also part of an exchange that came with learning. Some participants believed that contact with the REVEAL Study team might increase their likelihood of gaining access to new therapeutics for possible prevention:

> Albert wanted to reduce his risk for AD in order "to see if we could find out anything. And if there was something that they came up with that said, well, now, you know if you do this maybe, there would be a chance that you could reduce your possibility of having Alzheimer's. By all means, you'd try it."

> Kara inferred that prevention of AD for herself was important in the exchange for participation. "I got a flu shot today. I'd rather go with that and getting a vaccine, prevention being the key. If it could prevent it for me, was part of the deal—a big part."

> Peggy considered that she may have early access to potential therapeutics. "My thought at doing this was to know so that if something comes down the pipe that I could take that could circumvent it or prevent it, that I would be the first in line. That was my premise."

Need to know means a heightened sense of wanting information. Some participants expressed the need to know because of fear of developing AD or worrying about having symptoms that may mean already having early-onset AD:

Irene was frightened about inheriting AD. "But I got scared to death that I inherited this, and that's why I was anxious to get in the study and see. I wanted to know if I had the gene."

Frank described his "worrying" in his story of a "win-win" explanation. "And that's how I got involved in this, because my father was very sick and my stepmother got involved in this, so the family was involved. Well, I'm very much in the category of wanting to know. So I figured it was a win-win for me, because I was worrying some anyway without knowing. So for me, it was a fairly easy decision to want to do it."

Icarus already felt predestined. "Because I felt I was already doomed, so nothing that I could be told could be worse than what I already thought."

Cecelia wondered about having incipient symptoms of AD. "Then I became more focused on, obviously, my own probabilities. And I did what I tend to do, which is start seeking information. And a large amount of it—some of it—some of it, I think, is generated by an academic curiosity, which I've always had, whether it's personally driven or non-personally driven. And I realized that just going to a neurologist to do genetic testing was not going to do it. Yes. That, and, again, with the diagnosis and having been enveloped in my mother's Alzheimer's, her diagnosis, and also my focus, my cognizance of knowing—my memory has never been very strong. I'm bright, so I compensate. But my memory has never been very strong and my word finding, once I turned 50, seemed to become more pronounced. So I began thinking about, what does predisposition mean and, you know, what—I mean, obviously with my family members, onset was in the 70s. But what point do you start—you know, you begin thinking about, you know, am I—you know— am I predisposed? Am I—has it already begun but it's being-you know, buried?"

Model Development

We found that the core constructs, learning and altruism, were frequently coupled and illustrated an exchange of something of value (participation) between the REVEAL Study participant who has/had a parent

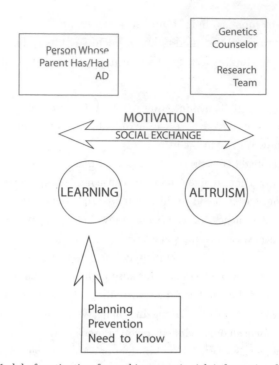

Figure 13.1. Model of motivation for seeking genetic risk information for AD

with AD and the REVEAL Study genetics counselor/research team (learning or information). Participants acted from a willingness and desire to support AD research while receiving something (learning or information) in exchange, something of value to self or children, including the potential for obtaining otherwise unavailable genetic information. This suggests an outright transaction between the study participant and the REVEAL Study team. This transaction is consistent with social exchange theory (Homans, 1961; Thibault and Kelley, 1959), which asserts that self-interested persons transact with other self-interested persons to accomplish individual goals that they cannot achieve alone. The model in figure 13.1 illustrates the social transaction of this reciprocal relationship.

The core constructs (altruism and learning) with the learning concepts (planning, prevention, and need to know) converge to describe motivation to participate in the REVEAL Study. The model describes the process of exchange identified in the stories. The exchange of altruism and learning operationalized the social process between the REVEAL Study's participants and the REVEAL Study's genetics counselor and research team members.

There was agreement between quantitative findings of motives for seeking testing in the REVEAL Study (Roberts et al., 2003, 2004) and the qualitative analysis of stories coded "why" in the REVEALED Project. Altruism, a core construct in the REVEALED Project, was strongly endorsed by 66 percent of the REVEALED participants. Participation in research provided something that was valued by the research team. Participants valued the construct of learning, with embedded concepts of planning, prevention, and need to know, which are consistent with strongly endorsed reasons for participation found in the REVEAL Study. "To arrange my personal affairs, to arrange my long-term care, to prepare my spouse or children for my illness, to do things sooner than I had planned to do them in the future," were ranked as numbers 2, 4, 5, and 7 respectively. Finding similar motives by using both quantitative and qualitative methods enhanced the reliability of both the REVEAL Study and REVEALED Project findings.

Conclusion

The REVEAL Study and subsequent REVEALED Project were the first empirical investigations to explore the motivation for obtaining risk assessment, the psychological consequences, and the changes made in health behaviors and insurance purchases after learning one's personal risk for AD from at-risk adult offspring of a parent with AD. Participants in these studies were actual stakeholders in near-real-world circumstances rather than ethicists or scientists using hypothetical scenarios. The five "negative" consensus papers, which recommended against APOE testing and disclosure for asymptomatic individuals, actually supported the need to go forward with research such as the REVEAL Study. Given the level of evidence at the time the consensus papers were published between 1995 and 1997, two to four years after the discovery of the role of the APOE gene as a risk factor for AD (Corder et al., 1993), it was appropriate then to argue against APOE testing used in a predictive manner. Now, empirically based evidence is available to help at-risk persons or patients, families, health care providers, researchers, and policy makers who previously have grappled with this issue.

At-risk persons and patients may benefit from reports that, although preliminary, suggest that the presence of the e4 allele may be associated with increased risk of converting from mild cognitive impairment to AD (Aggarwal et al., 2004; Petersen et al., 2005) and may be a possible marker for those who may benefit from specific therapeutics (Petersen et al., 2005). New discoveries of therapeutic agents to prevent or slow the progression of AD could add urgency to the need to identify at-risk individuals, making the use of genetic testing and disclosure clinically relevant. REVEAL participants were both generally satisfied with and unharmed by the experience of risk assessment for AD. The finding of "no significant changes in anxiety and depression scores between control and intervention participants" lowers the barrier against disclosure because of potential psychological harm (Roberts et al., 2005).

Family members face complex issues of potentially becoming long-term caregivers, being involved with a disease that affects all generations of a family, and being at increased risk for AD by virtue of being a first-degree relative of a person with AD. Larry addressed the concern of learning genetic risk for a disease when there is no current treatment for underlying pathology in these words: "I think it's very fitting with my personality that I like to understand things. And not that I could do anything about it, really, but I like to be understood and I like to understand." As people consider genetic testing for this complex, late-onset disease with no currently known preventative treatment, these findings can inform the way in which clinicians respond to family members' questions about future testing for their risk of developing AD.

Health care providers benefit from these findings in several ways. REVEAL Study data show that one year after disclosure, intervention group participants who were e4-positive were more likely to endorse AD-specific health behavior changes. Thus, there is the opportunity for capitalizing on this motivation and promoting positive health behaviors. Psychosocial interventions based on the conceptual approach of theories such as the health belief model (Becker, 1974) or self-efficacy theory (Bandura, 1986) can be used to promote healthy living habits that could protect the brain from AD. For example, head injury is a known risk factor for AD. So while everyone should wear seatbelts in cars and helmets when engaging in contact sports, it may be more important for persons who are e4-positive to do so. Likewise, while keeping blood pressure under control is important for everyone, it could turn out to be more important for persons at higher risk of developing AD.

The recently completed sequencing of the human genome and advances in basic science and technology will promote translational research in clinical genetics and lead to changes in health and disease paradigms. This in turn will generate many new opportunities for clinicians, who will incorporate genetic information and discoveries into patients' health care plans and who provide genetic health education. Health care providers should expect questions from family members about genetic testing (Schutte, 2006).

Researchers and policy makers are beneficiaries of these investigations in several ways. The model of the social transaction between the REVEAL Study's participants and research team illustrates not only reasons for seeking genetic susceptibility testing for AD but also for concurrent participation in a longitudinal research study. The revelation of complex and interwoven motivating factors can enhance the sensitivity of future scientists who conduct genetic research. Because some clinical trials of therapeutics for treating AD may be enriched by including persons who are e4-positive, knowing the potential for a social transaction between participants and the research team may serve to help in recruitment and maintaining participation in a longitudinal study. Policy makers may be interested in the impact of genetic susceptibility disclosure on health behaviors and insurance-purchasing behaviors.

The REVEAL Study and REVEALED Project provided answers to help persons at risk for AD or patients with AD, their family members, health care providers, and researchers. Results can serve to enhance the sensitivity of future scientists conducting genetic research and clinicians who are asked or will be asked, "Should I get tested?"

ACKNOWLEDGMENTS

Supported by the Alzheimer's Association (IRG-02-02213) (the REVEALED Project); Center for Nursing Excellence, Brigham and Women's Hospital, Boston, MA; National Institutes of Health (HG/AG-02213) (the REVEAL Study); Boston University Alzheimer's Disease Core Center (AG13846); Boston University General Clinical Research Center (RR00533); and Social Sciences and Humanities Research Council of Canada (SSHRC 205806).

REFERENCES

Aggarwal, N. T., R. Wilson, J. L. Bienias, E. Berry-Kravis, D. A. Evans, and D. A. Bennett. 2004. Risk factors for conversion from mild cognitive impairment to Alzheimer's disease. *Neurobiology of Aging* 25:S392.

Bandura, A. 1986. *Social Foundations of Thought and Action: A Social Cognitive Theory.* Englewood Cliffs, NJ: Prentice-Hall.

Becker, M. H. 1974. The health belief model and personal health behavior. *Health Education Monographs* 2:324–473.

Biesecker, B. B., and K. F. Peters. 2001. Process studies in genetic counseling: Peering into the black box. *American Journal of Medical Genetics* 106:191–98.

Blumer, H. 1969. *Symbolic Interactionism: Perspective and Method.* Englewood Cliffs, NJ: Prentice-Hall.

Brodaty, H., M. Conneally, S. Gauthier, C. Jennings, A. Lennox, and S. Lovestone. 1995. Consensus statement on predictive testing for Alzheimer disease. *Alzheimer Disease and Associated Disorders* 9:182–87.

Corder, E. H., A. M. Saunders, W. J. Strittmatter, D. E. Schmechel, P. C. Gaskell, G. W. Small, et al. 1993. Gene dose of apolipoprotein E type 4 allele and the risk of Alzheimer's disease in late onset families. *Science* 261:921–23.

Cupples, L. A., L. A. Farrer, A. D. Sadovnick, N. Relkin, P. Whitehouse, and R. C. Green. 2004. Estimating risk curves for first-degree relatives of patients with Alzheimer's disease: The REVEAL Study. *Genetics in Medicine* 6:192–96.

Cutler, S. J., and L. G. Hodgson. 2003. To test or not to test: Interest in genetic testing for Alzheimer's disease among middle-aged adults. *American Journal of Alzheimer's Disease and Other Dementias* 18:9–20.

Farrer, L. A., M. Brin, and L. Elsas. 1995. Statement on use of apolipoprotein E testing for Alzheimer disease. *Journal of the American Medical Association* 247:1627–29.

Glaser, B. G., and A. L. Strauss. 1967. *The Discovery of Grounded Theory: Strategies for Qualitative Research.* Chicago: Aldine.

Green, R. C. 2002. Risk assessment for Alzheimer's disease with genetic susceptibility testing: Has the moment arrived? *Alzheimer's Care Quarterly* 3:208–14.

Green, R. C., V. C. Clarke, N. J. Thompson, J. I. Woodard, and R. Letz. 1997. Early detection of Alzheimer disease: Methods, markers, and misgivings. *Alzheimer Disease and Associated Disorders* 11:1–5.

Homans, G. C. 1961. *Social Behavior: Its Elementary Forms.* New York: Harcourt Brace Jovanovich.

Hurley, A. C., R. Harvey, J. S. Roberts, C. Wilson-Chase, S. Lloyd, J. Prest, et al. 2005. Genetic susceptibility for Alzheimer's disease: Why did adult offspring seek testing? *American Journal of Alzheimer's Disease and Other Dementias* 20: 374–81.

Kearney, M. H. 2001. Levels and applications of qualitative research evidence. *Research in Nursing and Health* 24:145–53.

LaRusse, S., J. S. Roberts, T. M. Marteau, H. Katzen, E. L. Linnenbringer, M. Barber, et al. 2005. Genetic susceptibility testing versus family history–based risk assessment: Impact on perceived risk of Alzheimer disease. *Genetics in Medicine* 7:48–53.

Marteau, T. M., S. Roberts, S. LaRusse, and R. C. Green. 2005. Predictive genetic testing for Alzheimer's disease: Impact upon risk perception. *Risk Analysis* 25:397–404.

Miles, M. B., and A. M. Huberman. 1994. *Qualitative Data Analysis,* 2nd ed. Thousand Oaks, CA: SAGE Publications.

Pericak-Vance, M. A., M. P. Bass, L. H. Yamaoka, P. C. Gaskell, W. K. Scott, H. A. Terwedow, et al. 1997. Complete genomic screen in late-onset familial Alzheimer disease. *Journal of the American Medical Association* 278:1237–41.

Petersen, R. C., R. G. Thomas, M. Grundman, D. Bennett, R. Doody, S. Ferris, et al. 2005. Vitamin E and donepezil for the treatment of mild cognitive impairment. *New England Journal of Medicine* 352:2379–88.

Post, S. G., P. J. Whitehouse, R. H. Binstock, T. D. Bird, S. K. Eckert, L. A. Farrer, et al. 1997. The clinical introduction of genetic testing for Alzheimer disease: An ethical perspective. *Journal of the American Medical Association* 277:832–36.

Relkin, N. R. 1996. Apolipoprotein E genotyping in Alzheimer's disease. *Lancet* 347:1091–95.

Relkin, N. R., Y. J. Kwon, J. Tsai, and S. Gandy. 1996. The National Institute on Aging/Alzheimer's Association recommendations on the application of apolipoprotein E genotyping to Alzheimer's disease. *Annals of the New York Academy of Sciences* 802:149–76.

Rempusheski, V. F. 1999. Qualitative research and Alzheimer disease. *Alzheimer Disease and Associated Disorders* 13(suppl. 1).45–49.

Roberts, J. S. 2000. Anticipating response to predictive genetic testing for Alzheimer's disease: A survey of first-degree relatives. *Gerontologist* 40:43–52.

Roberts, J. S., S. A. LaRusse, H. Katzen, P. J. Whitehouse, M. Barber, S. G. Post, et al. 2003. Reasons for seeking genetic susceptibility testing among first-degree relatives of people with Alzheimer disease. *Alzheimer Disease and Associated Disorders* 17.00–93.

Roberts, J. S., M. Barber, T. M. Brown, L. A. Cupples, L. A. Farrer, S. A. LaRusse, et al. 2004. Who seeks genetic susceptibility testing for Alzheimer's disease? Findings from a multisite, randomized clinical trial. *Genetics in Medicine* 6:197–203.

Roberts, J. S., L. A. Cupples, N. R. Relkin, P. J. Whitehouse, and R. C. Green. 2005. Genetic risk assessment for adult children of people with Alzheimer's disease: The Risk Evaluation and Education for Alzheimer's Disease (REVEAL) Study. *Journal of Geriatric Psychiatry and Neurology* 18:250–55.

Roses, A. D. 1997. Genetic testing for Alzheimer disease: Practical and ethical issues. *Archives of Neurology* 54:1226–29.

Schutte, D. L. 2006. Alzheimer disease and genetics: Anticipating the questions. *American Journal of Nursing* 106:40–47.

Thibault, J. W., and H. H. Kelley. 1959. *The Social Psychology of Groups.* New York: Wiley.

Zick, C. D., C. J. Mathews, J. S. Roberts, R. Cook-Deegan, R. J. Pokorski, and R. C. Green. 2005. Genetic testing for Alzheimer's disease and its impact on insurance purchasing behavior. *Health Affairs* 24:483–90.

CHAPTER 14

Psychological Issues in Genetic Testing

J. SCOTT ROBERTS, PH.D.

Human genetics inhabits a volatile space at the intersection of
medicine, biology, corporate profits, law, government funding of
science, private insurance companies, genetic counseling
services . . . and popular culture.

—Alice Wexler, *Mapping Fate*

As discussed elsewhere in this volume, the implications of genetic research are profound and multifaceted. As Toni Miles points out in
chapter 15, genetic research has not yet yielded many findings that are
immediately relevant to primary care practitioners working with older
adults. For example, genetic testing is not yet available or recommended
for the most common diseases affecting older adults, often because of the
limited predictive value of current tests or a general lack of proven prevention options. However, there are many reasons to think that the "genetics revolution" may affect the care of older adults before long. Identification of genetic risk factors for diseases such as type 2 diabetes, Alzheimer
disease, Parkinson disease, and stroke raise the possibility that genetic
testing might ultimately be used to identify persons at high risk for these
common, late-life diseases (Saunders et al., 1993; Gretarsdottir et al., 2003;
Grant et al., 2006; Ozelius et al., 2006). As genetic links to late-onset disorders continue to be discovered, clinical care of older adults will increasingly involve consideration of gene testing for both older patients and
their blood relatives. Given the rapid pace of genetic research, practition-

ers and others involved with elder care would do well to educate themselves regarding the uses and limitations of genetic testing. This chapter
focuses on important issues to be considered in genetic testing, with a
particular emphasis on the psychological issues posed by such testing. A
general overview of clinical issues is provided, including a summary of
research findings to date and suggestions for future directions in the
field.

Issues to Consider
Test Characteristics

Genetic testing involves the analysis of human genetic material for heritable disorders. Purely genetic, or Mendelian, disorders are rare, but genetic factors often influence disease expression in more common disorders
(e.g., heart disease, cancer). Genetic testing may be conducted for disorders
with specific genetic causes that can be reliably identified, via procedures
such as biochemical assays and linkage testing (Roberts, 2001). DNA information can be obtained simply, through a blood sample or tissue sample
via a swab of the inner cheek. Genetic testing can be performed for either
diagnostic or predictive purposes. Of course, the predictive value of genetic
testing can vary greatly. Testing for autosomal dominant disorders (e.g.,
Huntington disease) can yield a nearly certain answer about whether or
not someone will develop the disease within a given timeframe. Susceptibility testing, on the other hand (e.g., for certain types of breast and colon
cancers), yields less definitive risk information. The certainty of test information has psychological implications, with regard to both initial interest
in testing and response to test results (Roberts, 2000).

Disease Characteristics

The characteristics of the disease for which genetic testing is being undertaken may have a marked impact on patients' psychological and behavioral response. The typical age of onset of a disease may influence the
types of issues that patients confront either before or after testing. For example, genetic test results for Huntington disease, which typically occurs
in midlife, can influence decisions on whether to marry or have children.
These issues might be less prominent, however, for those interested in genetic testing for late-onset Alzheimer disease, where retirement or insur-

TABLE 14.1
Summary of genetic test uptake rates, by disorder

Disorder	Usual age of onset	Type of testing	Effective prevention/ treatment options?	Estimated uptake rate (%)
Familial adenomatous polyposis	Adulthood	Predictive	Yes	85
Breast-ovarian cancer	Adulthood	Susceptibility	Yes	43
Hereditary nonpolyposis colorectal cancer	Adulthood	Susceptibility	Yes	30
Alzheimer disease	Late adulthood	Susceptibility	No	24
Cystic fibrosis	Childhood	Carrier screening	No	4–23
Huntington disease	Adulthood	Predictive	No	10

Source: Roberts et al., 2004.

ance planning issues may be a prime motivator (Roberts et al., 2003). Another factor influencing response to testing is the availability and effectiveness of treatments for a given disorder. As one would expect, interest in genetic testing tends to be much greater where the disorder can be prevented or treated. Table 14.1 shows how test uptake rates vary across various adult-onset diseases where interest in testing has been formally evaluated by research.

Who Should Provide Information?

An important question to consider is who should ultimately be providing genetic information to individuals and family members. Traditionally, genetic counselors have played this role, offering services in a relatively small number of specialty clinics, with time-intensive case preparation and nondirective counseling procedures. Yet there are concerns that the small number of genetic counselors could limit access to genetic services for growing numbers of patients. Others have argued that delivering risk information from susceptibility testing is well within the purview of standard physician-patient communication: because physicians discuss risk factors with patients on a routine basis, it has been suggested that to treat genetic risk factors differently would be a case of "genetic exceptionalism" (R. C. Green, 2002; M. J. Green et al., 2004). For these and other reasons, leaders in the field of genetic testing have called for a model of care emphasizing condensed protocols, increased collaboration with other health care professionals, and use of educational methods such as videotape and computer-based materials (Guttmacher, Jenkins, and Uhlmann, 2001). An interactive computer program has been developed for use in genetic counseling programs for breast cancer, with satisfactory patient education and satisfaction outcomes (M. J. Green et al., 2001a, 2001b). A potentially troubling development in the field is the emergence of "direct to consumer" marketing of genetic tests, which are generally unregulated and often offered without evidence of their safety and efficacy.

Individual Characteristics

The health psychology literature suggests many factors that are likely to influence response to genetic testing. For example, Miller developed the concept of health monitoring/blunting, which describes individual differences in information-seeking style under stress and the subsequent effects of these differences on health behavior (Miller, 1987). Monitors are individuals who in aversive situations tend to scan their environments for threat-relevant information, while blunters prefer to distract themselves from such information. This concept has been applied to genetic testing scenarios for breast cancer and Alzheimer disease (Lerman et al., 1994; Roberts, 2000).

It is also important to recognize that there may be notable individual differences in response to complex risk information, as the ability to understand principles of human genetics and statistical probability varies greatly across the population. Many studies have detailed the effects of patient "numeracy" on recall and comprehension of risk information (American Medical Association, 1999; Lipkus, Klein, and Rimer, 2001). The significance of patient literacy was highlighted in work on cancer genetic testing suggesting that up to one-third of participants lacked facility with basic probability and numerical concepts and often misinterpreted risk information (Schwartz et al., 1997). Many other studies have linked limited educational background with low interest in, and use of, genetic counseling (Lerman and Croyle, 1994; Geller et al., 1999; Glanz et al., 1999; Culver et al., 2001). It is therefore important to tailor educational approaches to patients' abilities to understand concepts involved in genetic risk assessment.

Finally, while much attention can be focused on the potential impact of "bad news" from a positive genetic test result, it appears that baseline psychological functioning is a better predictor of post-test response than test result itself. Research across several disorders has suggested that test-related distress, while significant at times, is usually transient if patients are provided proper post-test counseling (Marteau and Croyle, 1998). If test results match expectations, then even positive results for severe disorders are usually not overwhelming. However, if test results come "out of the blue" (as can happen in genetic screening programs), the psychological effects may be more pronounced (Roberts, 2001).

Research to Date

Genetic testing for adult-onset disorders has increasingly become a focus of behavioral research. This burgeoning literature has potential implications for clinical care of older adults. Summarized briefly here are findings across three classes of diseases for which genetic testing research has been conducted.

Huntington Disease

Huntington disease (HD) is the one adult-onset disorder in which protocols for presymptomatic, deterministic testing have been extensively used. Linkage analysis and gene identification have permitted highly accurate risk assessment for at-risk family members of persons with HD (Duyao et al., 1993, Huntington's Disease Collaborative Research Group, 1993). For the most part, HD predictive testing protocols include extensive and time-consuming highly structured pre- and post-test counseling guidelines, and HD testing is now routinely offered as a clinical service. A review of the literature about genetic testing for HD suggests the following: (1) Although initial interest in the test is high, uptake rates are relatively low (9–20%), with overrepresentation of women and more highly educated persons among those who choose to pursue testing. (2) People who choose to pursue testing generally show better psychological functioning than at-risk persons who decline testing. (3) People receiving results via linkage analysis (less certainty in the test) show better psychological outcomes than those receiving results through mutation detection (more certainty in the test). (4) Carriers experience greater transient distress in the weeks following disclosure of risk, but by six months both carriers and noncarriers are similar and generally without significant neg-

ative psychological effects of testing. (5) Psychological adjustment at baseline (e.g., level of depression or hopelessness) is a better predictor of post-
test adjustment than the test result itself (Meiser and Dunn, 2000).

Such research has shown that predictive testing for HD has had fewer
adverse outcomes than initially feared when it was introduced (Hayden,
2000). However, this not to say that test results are benign or recipients do
not sometimes experience significant distress as a result of undergoing
risk assessment. A worldwide assessment of adverse psychiatric outcomes
showed that around 1 percent of 4,527 HD test participants experienced
catastrophic events (i.e., attempted or completed suicide, psychiatric hospitalization) following testing; the vast majority of these participants had
received a positive test result (Almqvist et al., 1999). Even disclosure of
low risk can be stressful, if participants experience "survivor guilt" or re-
gret over irreversible decisions made with the assumption that they would
develop HD (Huggins et al., 1992). Furthermore, the impact of testing on
people without post-test counseling is unknown, suggesting that testing is
best offered in the context of available counseling resources. A study of
psychological outcomes seven to ten years following predictive testing for
HD suggests that distress levels are higher than in the two to three years
immediately following testing, presumably because individuals are closer
to the likely age of disease onset (Timman et al., 2004). This finding suggests a need for longer-term follow-up than is typically undertaken in
studies of the psychological impact of genetic testing.

Cancer

Susceptibility genes for various forms of cancer have been identified
such that genetic testing can now provide risk information for breast cancer, hereditary nonpolyposis colon cancer, familial adenomatous polypo-
sis, and colon cancer (Croyle et al., 1997; Lerman et al., 1996, 1999). Research in this area has focused on perceptions of cancer genetic testing
(Codori et al., 1999; Geller et al., 1999; Petersen et al., 1999; Press et al.,
2001; Welkenhuysen et al., 2001), the psychological impact of testing
(Aktan-Collan et al., 2000; Dorval et al., 2000; Esplen et al., 2001; Lodder
et al., 2001), risk communication issues (Croyle and Lerman, 1999; Daly
et al., 2001), cancer genetic knowledge and attitudes among health care
professionals (Geller et al., 1998; Cho et al., 1999; Escher and Sappino,

2000), and even the psychological impact of *not* pursuing genetic testing (Lerman et al., 1998).

A review of the literature suggested that genetic risk information did not necessarily result in changed health behaviors among those learning that they were at high risk for cancer (Marteau and Lerman, 2001). For example, testing for BRCA1/2 genes in women at risk for hereditary breast-ovarian cancer did not result in increased adherence to mammography at one-year follow-up (Lerman et al., 2000). These findings suggest that DNA information alone may not be sufficient to change patient behaviors regarding detection and risk management strategies.

A growing number of resources are now available both for clinicians and the lay public regarding cancer genetic testing. An excellent discussion of the psychological issues posed by genetic testing for cancer can be found in Andrea Farkas Patenaude's volume on the topic (Patenaude, 2004). In addition, the National Cancer Institute website includes an extensive listing of materials regarding cancer genetics, including general cancer genetics information, a directory of cancer genetics professionals, information on the genetics of specific cancers, and policy statement regarding genetic testing and genetic research (see www.nci.nih.gov/cancer info/prevention-genetics-causes/genetics). A notable policy statement is the American Society of Clinical Oncology's position paper on Genetic Testing for Cancer Susceptibility (American Society of Clinical Oncology, 2003).

Alzheimer Disease

Advances in genetic research on AD have raised the possibility of susceptibility testing for asymptomatic individuals (Roses, 1997; Masters and Beyreuther, 1998). The apolipoprotein E (APOE) e4 allele on chromosome 19 is a gene marker for AD whose impact on risk of AD has been widely confirmed (Farrer et al., 1997; Blacker and Tanzi, 1998; St. George-Hyslop, Farrer, and Goedert, 2000). While the presence of e4 allele(s) significantly increases risk of AD compared with other APOE genotypes (most estimates range from 316-fold), it is neither necessary nor sufficient to cause the disease (Farrer et al., 1997). APOE is thus distinct from the rare mutations that inevitably cause AD, typically with early onset (Karlinsky et al., 1994). Susceptibility testing for AD therefore differs in important ways from deterministic or predictive testing for disease-causing genes; it is relevant to a much larger at-risk population yet provides much less certain risk information (R. C. Green, 2002). This limitation, coupled with a general lack of treatment options for AD, has prompted several consensus statements cautioning against the premature introduction of susceptibility testing in asymptomatic individuals (Farrer et al., 1995; Relkin, 1996; Post et al., 1997). However, given treatment advances, potential patient demand, and clinical trials seeking "enriched" at-risk samples, there is a need to examine genetic risk assessment for AD in a research context (McConnell et al., 1998; R. C. Green, 2002).

The federally funded Risk Evaluation and Education for Alzheimer's Disease (REVEAL) Study is the first randomized controlled trial (RCT) designed to evaluate the impact of risk assessment, using APOE genotype disclosure, for AD. The study protocol was developed by a team of experts in the fields of neurology, genetics, genetic counseling, psychology, and bioethics. Protocol development was overseen and approved by an External Advisory Board and institutional review boards at each original study site (Boston, New York, Cleveland). All study participants were adult children of a person with clinically diagnosed and/or autopsy-confirmed AD. Before enrollment in the RCT, participants attended a formal Education Session conducted by the site's genetic counselor, where information about AD, genetic testing, and the study protocol was provided using a slide show presentation. Personalized risk information that incorporated gender, family history, and APOE genotype was disclosed to participants; risk estimates ranged from 13 to 57 percent and were based on a large-scale genetic epidemiology research based at Boston University (Cupples et al., 2004). A total of 162 persons participated in the study's first clinical trial, and findings published to date have focused on the following topics: (1) participants' reasons for pursuing genetic testing for AD (Roberts et al., 2003); (2) factors associated with test uptake (Roberts et al., 2004); (3) the impact of genetic testing on risk perceptions (LaRusse et al., 2005; Marteau et al., 2005); and (4) the impact of genetic testing on insurance behavior (Zick et al., 2005). Preliminary findings suggest that genetic information did not generally have adverse psychological consequences for participants, providing the basis for a second clinical trial examining a briefer, more clinically feasible risk assessment protocol (Roberts et al., 2005).

Conclusion

A burgeoning research literature is addressing numerous topics regarding psychological and behavioral response to genetic testing. However, the field is still relatively young, and much work remains to be done. One area for improvement concerns research methodology. Outcome measures have been criticized as not being sensitive enough to assess the psychological impact of genetic testing. New measures, such as the Multidimensional Impact of Cancer Risk Assessment (MICRA), are being employed to assess the impact of genetic testing (Cella et al., 2002). In addition, more sophisticated measures are being used to assess not only the outcomes of genetic testing and counseling but also its process. The Roter Interaction Analysis System is a well-validated coding method to analyze patient-provider interactions that has been used widely over the past 25 years and that has been adapted for use in genetic counseling research (Roter et al., 1997; Ellington et al., 2005).

Another future direction for research in this area is to increase sample diversity, as racial and ethnic minorities have typically been underrepresented, as have people of lower socioeconomic status. The REVEAL Study has partnered with the Howard University National Human Genome Center to examine issues involved in African Americans' experience of genetic risk assessment for Alzheimer disease. Finally, an interesting area for future research concerns the topic of *pleiotropy:* that is, recognizing that individual genes may affect more than one organ system and thereby increase susceptibility for multiple disorders at once. The APOE gene is a case in point, as the e4 allele serves as a risk factor not only for Alzheimer disease but also for certain types of cardiovascular disease (Olichney et al., 1997; Gerdes et al., 2000; Lahoz et al., 2001). Learning how to communicate about the risks posed by particular pleiotropic genes may represent an increasingly common challenge for clinicians in coming decades. Indeed, as genetic research increasingly informs clinical care of older adults, it will be important to consider the ethical, legal, and social implications of such research. As Richards and Marteau commented, "Social scientists have an important role to play in conducting research on developments in the new human genetics. We should not, and probably cannot anyway, stop further technical developments in the field. But we must not be passive and let the technological tail wag the societal dog. We must join the debate and help to negotiate the kind of future we all want" (Marteau and Richards, 1996, 353).

ACKNOWLEDGMENTS

Supported by NIH grants RO1-HG/AG02213 (the REVEAL Study), P30-AG13846 (Boston University Alzheimer's Disease Core Center), and M01-RR00533 (Boston University General Clinical Research Center).

REFERENCES

Aktan-Collan, K., J. P Mecklin, A. de la Chapelle, P. Peltomaki, A. Uutela, and H. Kaariainen. 2000. Evaluation of a counseling protocol for predictive genetic testing for hereditary non-polyposis colorectal cancer. *Journal of Medical Genetics* 37:108–13.

Almqvist, E., M. Bloch, R. Brinkman, D. Craufurd, and M. Hayden. 1999. A worldwide assessment of the frequency of suicide, suicide attempts, or psychiatric hospitalization after predictive testing for Huntington disease. *American Journal of Human Genetics* 64:1293–1304.

American Medical Association. 1999. Ad hoc committee on health literacy for the council on scientific affairs, American Medical Association. *Journal of the American Medical Association*. 281:552–57.

American Society of Clinical Oncology. 2003. American Society of Clinical Oncology policy statement update: Genetic testing for cancer susceptibility. *Journal of Clinical Oncology* 21(12):1–10.

Blacker, D., and R. Tanzi. 1998. The genetics of Alzheimer disease: Current status and future prospects. *Archives of Neurology* 55:294–96.

Cella, D., C. Hughes, A. Peterman, C. H. Chang, B. N. Peshkin, L. Wenzel, et al. 2002. A brief assessment of concerns associated with genetic testing for cancer: The Multidimensional Impact of Cancer Risk Assessment (MICRA) questionnaire. *Health Psychology* 21:564–72.

Cho, M. K., P. Sankar, P. R. Wolpe, and L. Godmilow. 1999. Commercialization of BRCA1/2 testing: Practitioner awareness and use of a new genetic test. *American Journal of Medical Genetics* 83:157–63.

Codori, A. M., G. M. Petersen, D. L. Miglioretti, E. K. Larkin, M. T. Bushey, C. Young, et al. 1999. Attitudes toward colon cancer gene testing: Factors predicting test uptake. *Cancer Epidemiology, Biomarkers, and Prevention* 8:345–51.

Croyle, R. T., and C. Lerman. 1999. Risk communication in genetic testing for cancer susceptibility. *Journal of the National Cancer Institute* 25:59–66.

Croyle, R. T., K. R. Smith, J. R. Botkin, B. Baty, and J. Nash. 1997. Psychological responses to BRCA1 mutation testing: Preliminary findings. *Health Psychology* 16:63–72.

Culver, J., W. Burke, Y. Yasui, S. Durfy, and N. Press. 2001. Participation in breast cancer genetic counseling: The influence of educational level, ethnic background, and risk perception. *Journal of Genetic Counseling* 10:215–31.

Cupples, L. A., L. Farrer, D. Sadovnick, N. Relkin, P. Whitehouse, and R. C. Green. 2004. Estimating risk curves for first-degree relatives of patients with Alzheimer's disease: The REVEAL Study. *Genetic Medicine* 6(4):192–96.

Daly, M. B., A. Barsevick, S. M. Miller, R. Buckman, J. Costalas, S. Montgomery, et al. 2001. Communicating genetic test results to the family: A six step, skills building strategy. *Family and Community Health* 24(3):13–26.

Dorval, M., A. F. Patenaude, K. A. Schneider, S. A. Kieffer, L. DiGianni, K. J. Kalkbrenner, et al. 2000. Anticipated versus actual emotional reactions to disclosure of results of genetic tests for cancer susceptibility: Findings from p53 and BRCA1 testing programs. *Journal of Clinical Oncology* 18:2135–42.

Duyao, M., C. Ambrose, R. Myers, A. Novelletto, F. Persichetti, M. Frontali, et al. 1993. Trinucleotide repeat length instability and age of onset in Huntington's disease. *Nature Genetics* 4:387–92.

Ellington, L., D. Roter, W. N. Dudley, B. J. Baty, R. Upchurch, S. Larson, et al. 2005. Communication analysis of BRCA1 genetic counseling. *Journal of Genetic Counseling* 14:377–86.

Escher, M., and A. P. Sappino. 2000. Primary care physicians' knowledge and attitudes toward genetic testing for breast-ovarian cancer predisposition. *Annals of Oncology* 11:1131–35.

Esplen, M. J., L. Madlensky, K. Butler, W. McKinnon, B. Bapat, J. Wong, et al. 2001. Motivations and psychosocial impact of genetic testing for HNPCC. *American Journal of Medical Genetics* 103:9–15.

Farrer, L. A., M. F. Brin, L. Elsas, A. Goate, J. Kennedy, R. Mayeux, et al. 1995. Statement on use of apolipoprotein E testing for Alzheimer disease. *Journal of the American Medical Association* 274:1627–29.

Farrer, L. A., L. A. Cupples, J. L. Haines, B. Hyman, W. A. Kukull, R. Mayeux, et al. 1997. Effects of age, sex, and ethnicity on the association between apolipoprotein E genotype and Alzheimer disease: A meta-analysis. *Journal of the American Medical Association* 278:1349–56.

Geller, G., B. A. Bernhardt, T. Doksum, K. J. Helzlsouer, P. Wilcox, and N. A. Holtzman. 1998. Decision-making about breast cancer susceptibility testing: How similar are the attitudes of physicians, nurse practitioners, and at-risk women? *Journal of Clinical Oncology* 16:2868–76.

Geller, G., T. Doksum, B. A. Bernhardt, and S. A. Metz. 1999. Participation in breast cancer susceptibility testing protocols: Influence of recruitment source, altruism, and family involvement on women's decisions. *Cancer Epidemiology, Biomarkers, and Prevention* 8:377–83.

Gerdes, L. U., C. Gerdes, K. Kervinen, M. Savolainen, I. C. Klausen, P. S. Hansen, et al. 2000. The apolipoprotein epsilon4 allele determines prognosis and the effect on prognosis of simvastatin in survivors of myocardial infarction: A substudy of the Scandinavian simvastatin survival study. *Circulation* 101: 1366 71.

Glanz, K., J. Grove, C. Lerman, C. Gotay, and L. LeMarchand. 1999. Correlates of intentions to obtain genetic counseling and colorectal cancer gene testing among at-risk relatives from three ethnic groups. *Cancer Epidemiology, Biomarkers, and Prevention* 8:329–36.

Grant, S. F. A., G. Thorleifsson, I. Reynisdottir, R. Benediktsson, A. Manolescu, J. Sainz, et al. 2006. Variant of transcription factor 7-like 2 (TCF7L2) gene confers risk of type 2 diabetes. *Nature Genetics,* online publication, 1–4.

Green, M. J., B. B. Biesecker, A. M. McInerney, D. Mauger and N. Fost. 2001a. An interactive computer program can effectively educate patients about genetic testing for breast cancer susceptibility. *American Journal of Medical Genetics* 103:16–23.

Green, M. J., A. M. McInerney, B. B. Biesecker, and N. Fost. 2001b. Education about genetic testing for breast cancer susceptibility: Patient preferences for a computer program or genetic counselor. *American Journal of Medical Genetics* 103: 24–31.

Green, M. J., S. K. Petersen, M. Baker, G. R. Harper, L. C. Friedman, W. S. Rubinstein, et al. 2004. Effect of a computer-based decision aid on knowledge, perceptions, and intentions about genetic testing for breast cancer susceptibility: A randomized controlled trial. *Journal of the American Medical Association* 292: 442–52.

Green, R. C. 2002. Genetic susceptibility testing for Alzheimer's disease: Has the moment arrived? *Alzheimer's Care Quarterly* 3:208–14.

Gretarsdottir, S., G. Thorleifsson, S. T. Reynisdottir, A. Manolescu, S. Jonsdottir, T. Jonsdottir, et al. 2003. The gene encoding phosphodiesterase 4D confers risk of ischemic stroke. *Nature Genetics* 35:131–38.

Guttmacher, A. E., J. Jenkins, and W. R. Uhlmann. 2001. Genomic medicine: Who will practice it? A call to open arms. *American Journal of Medical Genetics* 106:216–22.

Hayden, M. R. 2000. Predictive testing for Huntington's disease: The calm after the storm. *Lancet* 356:216–22.

Huggins, M., M. Bloch, S. Wiggins, S. Adams, O. Suchowersky, M. Trew, et al. 1992. Predictive testing for Huntington's disease in Canada: Adverse effects and unexpected results in those receiving a decreased risk. *American Journal of Medical Genetics* 42:508–15.

Huntington's Disease Collaborative Research Group. 1993. A novel gene containing a trinucleotide repeat that is expanded and unstable on Huntington's disease chromosomes. *Cell* 72:971–83.

Karlinsky, H., A. D. Sadovnick, M. M. Burgess, S. Langlois, M. R. Hayden, and J. M. Berg. 1994. Issues in molecular genetic testing of individuals with suspected early-onset familial Alzheimer's disease. *Alzheimer Disease and Associated Disorders* 8(2):116–25.

Lahoz, C., E. J. Schaefer, L. A. Cupples, P. W. F. Wilson, D. Levy, D. Osgood, et al. 2001. Apolipoprotein E genotype and cardiovascular disease in the Framingham Heart Study. *Atherosclerosis* 154:529–37.

LaRusse, S. A., J. S. Roberts, T. Marteau, H. Katzen, E. Linnenbringer, M. Barber, et al. 2005. Genetic susceptibility testing versus family history–based risk assessment: Impact on perceived risk of Alzheimer's disease. *Genetics in Medicine* 7:48–53.

Lerman, C., and R. T. Croyle. 1994. Psychological issues in genetic testing for breast cancer susceptibility. *Archives of Internal Medicine* 154:609–16.

Lerman, C., M. Daly, A. Masny, and A. Balshem. 1994. Attitudes about genetic testing for breast-ovarian cancer susceptibility. *Journal of Clinical Oncology* 12:843–50.

Lerman, C., C. Hughes, J. L. Benkendorf, B. Biesecker, J. Kerner, J. Willison, et al. 1999. Racial differences in testing motivation and psychological distress following pretest education for BRCA1 gene testing. *Cancer Epidemiology, Biomarkers, and Prevention* 8:61–67.

Lerman, C., C. Hughes, R. T. Croyle, and D. Main. 2000. Prophylactic surgery decisions and surveillance practices one year following BRCA1/2 testing. *Preventive Medicine* 31:75–80.

Lerman, C., C. Hughes, S. J. Lemon, D. Main, C. Snyder, C. Durham, et al. 1998. What you don't know can hurt you: Adverse psychologic effects in members of BRCA1-linked and BRCA2-linked families who decline genetic testing. *Journal of Clinical Oncology* 16:1650–54.

Lerman, C., S. Narod, K. Schulman, C. Hughes, A. Gomez-Caminero, G. Bonney, et al. 1996. BRCA1 testing in families with hereditary breast ovarian cancer: A prospective study of patient decision making and outcomes. *Journal of the American Medical Association* 275:1885–92.

Lipkus, I. M., W. M. Klein, and B. K. Rimer. 2001. Communicating breast cancer risks to women using different formats. *Cancer Epidemiology, Biomarkers, and Prevention* 10:895–98.

Lodder, L., P. G. Frets, R. W. Trijsburg, E. J. Meijers-Heijboer, J. G. Klijn, H. J. Duivenvoorden, et al. 2001. Psychological impact of receiving a BRCA1/BRCA2 test result. *American Journal of Medical Genetics* 98:15–24.

Marteau, T. M., and R. T. Croyle. 1998. The new genetics: Psychological responses to genetic testing. *British Medical Journal* 316:693–96.

Marteau, T. M., and C. Lerman. 2001. Genetic risk and behavioural change. *British Medical Journal* 322:1056–59.

Marteau, T. M., and M. Richards. 1996. *The Troubled Helix: Social and Psychological Implications of the New Human Genetics.* New York: Cambridge University Press.

Marteau, T. M., J. S. Roberts, S. A. LaRusse, and R. C. Green. 2005. Predictive genetic testing for Alzheimer's disease: Impact upon risk perception. *Risk Analysis* 25:397–404.

Masters, C. L., and K. Beyreuther. 1998. Science, medicine, and the future: Alzheimer's disease. *British Medical Journal* 316:446–48.

McConnell, L. M., B. A. Koenig, H. T. Greely, and T. A. Raffin. 1998. Genetic testing and Alzheimer disease: Has the time come? *Nature Medicine* 5:757–60.

Moiscr, D., and S. Dunn. 2000. Psychological impact of genetic testing for Huntington's disease: An update of the literature. *Journal of Neurology, Neurosurgery, and Psychiatry* 69:574–78.

Miller, S. M. 1987. Monitoring and blunting: Validation of a questionnaire to assess styles of information seeking under threat. *Journal of Personality and Social Psychology* 52:345–53.

Olichney, J., M. Sabbagh, C. Hofstetter, D. Galasko, M. Grundman, R. Katzman, et al. 1997. The impact of apolipoprotein E4 on cause of death in Alzheimer's disease. *Neurology* 49:76–81.

Ozelius, L. J., G. Senthil, R. Saunders-Pullman, E. Ohmann, A. Deligtisch, M. Tagliati, et al. 2006. LRRK2 G2019S as a cause of Parkinson's disease in Ashkenazi Jews. *New England Journal of Medicine* 354:424–25.

Patenaude, A. F. 2004. *Genetic testing for cancer: Psychological approaches for helping patients and families.* Washington, DC: American Psychological Association.

Petersen, G. M., E. Larkin, A. M. Codori, C. Y. Wang, S. V. Booker, J. Bacon, et al. 1999. Attitudes toward colon cancer gene testing: Survey of relatives of colon cancer patients. *Cancer Epidemiology, Biomarkers, and Prevention* 8:337–44.

Post, S. G., P. J. Whitehouse, R. H. Binstock, T. D. Bird, S. K. Eckert, L. A. Farrer, et al. 1997. The clinical introduction of genetic testing for Alzheimer's disease: An ethical perspective. *Journal of the American Medical Association* 277:832–36.

Press, N. A., Y. Yasui, S. Reynolds, S. J. Durfy, and W. Burke. 2001. Women's interest in genetic testing for breast cancer susceptibility may be based on unrealistic expectations. *American Journal of Medical Genetics* 99:99–110.

Relkin, N. 1996. NIA/Alzheimer's Association Working Group: Apolipoprotein E genotyping in Alzheimer's disease. *Lancet* 347:1091–95.

Roberts, J. S. 2000. Anticipating response to predictive genetic testing for Alzheimer's disease: A survey of first-degree relatives. *Gerontologist* 40:43–52.

Roberts, J. S. 2001. Genetic testing. In *Encyclopedia of Care of the Elderly*, ed. M. Mezey. Pp. 298–300. New York: Springer.

Roberts, J. S., M. Barber, T. M. Brown, L. A. Cupples, L. A. Farrer, S. A. LaRusse, et al. 2004. Who seeks genetic susceptibility testing for Alzheimer's disease? Findings from a multisite, randomized clinical trial. *Genetics in Medicine* 6: 197–203.

Roberts, J. S., L. A. Cupples, N. Relkin, P. J. Whitehouse, and R. C. Green. 2005. Genetic risk assessment for adult children of people with Alzheimer's disease: The Risk Evaluation and Education for Alzheimer's Disease (REVEAL) Study. *Journal of Geriatric Psychiatry and Neurology* 18:250–55.

Roberts, J. S., S. A. LaRusse, H. Katzen, P. J. Whitehouse, M. Barber, S. G. Post, et al. 2003. Reasons for seeking genetic susceptibility testing among first-degree relatives of people with Alzheimer's disease. *Alzheimer Disease and Associated Disorders* 17(2):86–93.

Roses, A. D. 1997. Genetic testing for Alzheimer disease: Practical and ethical issues. *Archives of Neurology* 54:1226–29.

Roter, D. L., M. Stewart, S. Putnam, M. Lipkin, W. Stiles, and T. Innui. 1997. Communication patterns of primary care physicians. *Journal of the American Medical Association* 270:350–55.

Saunders, A. M., W. J. Strittmatter, D. Schmechel, D., P. H. St. George-Hyslop, M. A. Pericak-Vance, S. H. Joo, et al. 1993. Association of apolipoprotein E allele e4 with late-onset familial and sporadic Alzheimer's disease. *Neurology* 43:1467–72.

Schwartz, L. M., S. Woloshin, W. C. Black, and H. G. Welch. 1997. The role of numeracy in understanding the benefit of screening mammography. *Annals of Internal Medicine* 127:966–72.

St. George-Hyslop, P. H., L. A. Farrer, and M. Goedert. 2000. Alzheimer disease and the fronto-temporal dementias: Diseases with cerebral deposition of fibrillar proteins. In *Molecular and Metabolic Basis of Inherited Disease,* 8th ed. Vol. 4, pp. 5785–5899. Columbus, OH: McGraw-Hill.

Timman, R., R. Roos, A. Maat-Kievit, and A. Tibben. 2004. Adverse effects of predictive testing for Huntington disease underestimated: Long-term effects 7–10 years after the test. *Health Psychology* 23(2):189–97.

Welkenhuysen, M., G. Evers-Kiebooms, M. Decruyenaere, E. Claes, and L. Denayer. 2001. A community based study on intentions regarding predictive testing for hereditary breast cancer. *Journal of Medical Genetics* 38:540–47.

Wexler, A. 1996. *Mapping Fate: A Memoir of Family, Risk, and Genetic Research.* Berkeley: University of California Press.

Zick, C. D., C. Matthews, J. S. Roberts, R. Cook-Deegan, R. J. Pokorski, and R. C. Green. 2005. Genetic susceptibility testing for Alzheimer's disease and its impact on insurance purchasing behavior. *Health Affairs* 24:483–90.

Genotype, Phenotype, and Primary Care

Why the New Genetics Technology Is Not Ready for Primary Care

TONI P. MILES, M.D., PH.D.

Public health and genetics professionals who advocate the use of genetics in primary care tout its ability to identify persons with elevated risk of disease. These advocates argue that persons aged 65 years or older may especially benefit from genetics technology because the diseases that are responsible for almost 70 percent of all deaths for this age group are either underlying cardiovascular disease or cancer (Bernstein et al., 2003), and genes that increase an individual's risk of developing these disorders have been identified (Lindor and Greene, 1998; Winkelman et al., 2000). There is considerable enthusiasm among governmental and professional entities for this point of view. Awareness of family history and personal genetic susceptibility appears to hold so much promise that the U.S. Surgeon General's Office launched a Family History Initiative (www.hhs.gov/familyhistory). This website is designed to assist families in developing a health portrait so as to identify familial aggregations of disease. The National Coalition for Health Professional Education in Genetics (NCHPEG) developed a set of core competencies in genetics that it considers essential for all health care professionals (www.nchpeg.org/eduresources/core/core .asp) and an electronic training module in genetics, common disorders, and the implications of these new risk factors for the management of disease by primary care providers. This program includes case studies (thrombophilia, colorectal cancer), training in the fundamentals of genetics, and an approach to applying genomics to the prevention and management of disease as well as a discussion of the associated ethical, legal, and social implications.

Primary care providers have responded to this explosion of information by asking the following question: Among patients who already have a disease, how does knowing that they have a genetic susceptibility alter my medical management of their current condition? Consider the case if the disorder were diabetes. The majority of patients with type 2 diabetes are not seen consistently by a primary care physician until *after* the disease develops. In other words, most physicians do not see a patient with any regularity until the disease process reaches the threshold where clinical markers are detected. Persons with undiagnosed diabetes typically do not seek medical care until they have one of the following complaints: "I am thirsty and tired all the time," or "I have difficulty attaining or maintaining an erection," or "I just don't feel like myself." The complaint is evaluated, and an elevation in blood sugar is identified, which may or may not be accompanied by elevated lipids, elevated blood pressure, or elevated body weight. At this stage, knowing genetic susceptibility does not alter medical management for the patient.

What if a clinician with a public health orientation wanted to work with the family of the patient described above? He or she might ask the genetics professional this question: Does knowing that someone has a strong family history of type 2 diabetes change my approach to prevention or delay the onset of disease in other family members? Right now diet, exercise, and weight control are the only approaches available for physicians to reduce the risk of developing diabetes among family members who do not have the full-blown clinical syndrome. In other words, having genotype information available at the moment of family counseling does not change medical strategy. What might be useful would be to know if the knowledge of genetic susceptibility to type 2 diabetes would change familial acceptance of modifications in diet and physical activity habits. That important and highly relevant question is beyond the scope of this chapter. My focus will be on the primary care provider, the aged patient, and the potential utility of the new genetics technology for improving health care delivered to the individual.

What do we mean when we say primary care? Primary care is medical treatment provided during "first contact" in the health care system. Patients at this stage are undifferentiated (i.e., do not have a diagnostic label). The process of responding to the patient's problem includes an interview process as well as the application of directed medical technology to gather information. If the patient is seeking relief from suffering, then family history and genetic testing might improve the accuracy of diagnostic labeling. However, most of the common conditions of aging do not require genetic testing as a part of the diagnostic protocol. For example, diagnosis of osteoporosis and related fractures does not require testing for high-risk genes indicating a skeletal, endocrine, or vitamin metabolism etiology. It is likely that most third-party health insurance payers would deny claims for administration of genetic tests under these circumstances. Altruism could be used to make a strong case for genetic testing for the benefit of younger family members, but the individual (or the family) would still bear the economic burden for such testing and for most preventative measures that might follow. If the older adult has sufficient financial resources, then obtaining the information would be viewed as trading health for wealth. This practice has been described by economists in studies of intergenerational transfer of wealth (Shea, Miles, and Hayward, 1996). In the same way that inheritance of monetary resources and property benefit children and grandchildren, one could argue that a clear identification of high-risk genes could also be a legacy.

Primary care also includes health promotion, disease prevention, and management of chronic disease. In the United States, the U.S. Task Force for Preventive Services (USTFPS), a panel of experts in primary care and prevention, is responsible for promoting clinical guidelines for the application of treatments in medical practice. These clinical guidelines are based on a determination of the benefits and harms of screening/testing/treating illnesses. The final determination of clinical utility is a result of an extensive search of the medical literature using the Cochrane Library database of clinical trials, other reference lists, reviews, and websites. The Agency for Healthcare Research and Quality (AHRQ) maintains a database of evidence-based clinical practice guidelines, the National Guideline Clearing House, usually developed by professional organizations such as a medical specialty society, government agency, health care organization, or health plan. Although many genes have been identified in clinical studies of high-risk families as having a large influence on, say, the probability of developing cancer, there is insufficient evidence of the utility of screening for any of these genes in routine clinical practice. A search of the USTFPS, AHRQ's National Guideline Clearing House, and the Canadian Task Force on Preventive Care produced only two clinical guidelines addressing the issue of genetic screening for cancer: one on breast/ovarian cancer (Nelson et al., 2005) and the other on colorectal cancer (Canadian Task Force on Preventive Health Care, 2001). In the case of colorectal cancer, there is not sufficient evidence to support routine genetic screening in the general population. For breast and ovarian cancer, the reviewers indicate that there is a lack of evidence to balance benefits against harms of genetic screening in the general population. In the absence of direct evidence, Nelson and colleagues develop an estimate of the magnitude of potential benefits and adverse effects for screening of the general population. They take the further step of stratifying the population by average, moderate, and high risk of mutations based on family history. How are the risks and benefits of cancer screening to be reconciled? After starting with a sample of 100,000 women containing 431 high-risk women imbedded in the population, an estimated 16 cases of breast cancer would be prevented by implementation of routine genetic screening of all primary care patients. Neither article specifically addresses the implications of genetic testing for the care of the older adult.

Research such as this does not fully address real-world questions. How are primary care clinic samples different from genetics study samples? How do gene mutations strongly predict disease when measured in cancer patients but fail to show an association when studied in the general population? These are important questions for patients who carry the high-risk genes as well as for those who don't. These seemingly discordant results can be attributable to the mathematics of clinical test performance assessment. The results of these calculations are strongly influenced by the amount of background disease in the test sample. Conceptually this is an estimate of the probability that a test can detect a case of disease. The more sensitive the test, the fewer cases are missed. Sound confusing? It can be, especially when the background rates of "true" cases are different for each test population. Consider the scenario of a population where everyone is a "true" genetic case. You are standing by a window and watching people come and go. Your "genetic" test consists of throwing rocks at people. The hypothesis is that only persons with the clinically important gene will be hit by a rock because the underlying genetic defect makes them somehow attractive to rocks! Under this absurd scenario, rock throwing is a very sensitive test because 100 percent of the time it will hit someone with a disease directly attributable to their genetic makeup. There are two types of people that we could add to the sample outside our window. We could add people who carry the gene but do not manifest the disease. We could also add people who have the disease but do not have the gene. In both cases, the ability of our rock test to detect genetically informative cases would decline. The current state of genetic screening in the general population does not function much better than throwing rocks.

Genetic variation and its relationship to disease occurrence among primary care patient panels are phenomena that have not been well studied. Understanding the intersection between these two phenomena has the potential for improving our understanding of the application of routine genetic screening in primary care. Figure 15.1 illustrates how individual variation in a clinical measure can be complicated by clustering within a primary care panel. The graph was developed using data from our studies of primary care clinics. On the y-axis, values for a test (CLOX1 Research Score) were plotted. A patient can score between 0 and 14, and the larger the number, the better the performance on the test. Each box represents a separate clinic site with no overlap between patients. The black line in the middle of each box is the median score for each clinic. The length of the box shows the range of scores for 66 percent of patients measured at each clinic. The line passing through each box represents the range of scores for 95 percent of all patients in the clinic. The dots and stars show individual patients who fall outside of their clinic's range.

There are several points to be made with this graph. First, although the average values for our test are not significantly different across clinics *A* through *M*, there is clinically significant variation within the panels. Any patient with a score of 9 or less is considered to have clinically important disease. Clinics *A* and *F* look identical, but the scores of the outliers are quite different. Next, the wider the range of values, the greater effect it has on whether an individual is viewed as being an "unusual" clinical case. For example, the five "outlier" patients in clinic *E* would not be unusual in clinic *A*. Finally, although the measured values of the worst cases are identical in clinics *F*, *J*, *K*, and *L*, the ages of the involved patients is quite

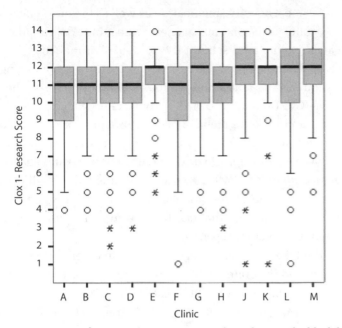

Figure 15.1. Variation in disease rating score across clinical sites. The black line shows median value for each location. The box encompasses 66 percent of all scores for the location. The dots represent scores outside of the 95 percent range.

different: 49 years, 22 years, and 82 years, respectively (data not shown). This suggests that although the diagnostic labels are the same, the underlying process may not be similar at all. When applied to the problem of heritable diseases, this example shows us that there is considerable heterogeneity in underlying clinical diseases that may not always be appreciated.

Is there any aspect of the new genetics technology that might be applied to benefit in a general patient population? Pharmacogenetic tests represent a special category of genetic tests that will likely play an important role in primary care in the near future. There are three main potential uses of genetic tests in guiding individualized drug therapy that are especially important for older adults. These tests can be used to avoid serious adverse events due to individual, metabolic idiosyncrasies. For example, most drugs implicated in creating the life-threatening cardiac dysrhythmia QT interval prolongation can be linked to pharmacogenetic identifiable enzymes and genes (Caldwell, 2001). Older adults are the group with the highest rates of adverse drug reactions, and any test that can prevent these problems are well worth the expense.

Finding the most effective medication as well as the most effective dose are other advantages of pharmacogenetic screening. Depression is quite common among older adults, but if it is untreated or ineffectively treated, it is also associated with premature mortality. Appropriate dosing of the antidepressant medications amitriptyline and nortriptyline can be refined by measuring CY2D6 and CYD2C19 activity rates (Steimer et al., 2004). Persons who are extensive metabolizers require greater doses to achieve mood improvement. Currently the most complete discussion of pharmacogenetics has been developed with support from the Wellcome Trust. *My Very Own Medicine: What Must I Know?* presents a thorough discussion of all of these issues and more (Melzer et al., 2003). Its stated goal is the presentation of information that can be used to make policy guiding the implementation of pharmacogenetics.

What will it take for primary care providers to embrace the new genetics technology and integrate it into routine care? This is probably the most complex question of all that could be asked. Certainly the science behind identification of genetic polymorphisms in drug metabolism (P450 system) demonstrates a clear and compelling case for inclusion (Ingelman-Sundberg, 2004). One gene alone, CYP2D6, is involved in the metabolism of almost 70 percent of drugs used in practice. Two studies have explored primary care provider attitudes toward the new genetics. One author argues that provider resistance to implementation of this technology is primarily related to a lack of education about its benefits (Watson et al., 1999). Robbins and Metcalfe (2004) present an opposing view. They argue that resistance is not based in a "cognitive deficit" (i.e., that there is a lack of understanding of the technology). Instead, practitioners expressed the concern that this information does not change practice. Although it is not expressed directly in surveys of primary care providers, there is also the issue of medical liability and pharmacogenomics (Palmer, 2003). Currently, there are no clinical guidelines for responding to these data, so the assessment of the risk-benefit of knowing and acting on that knowledge falls squarely into the lap of the provider.

The U.S. population is derived from countries drawn from across the globe. While each group has similar major metabolic pathways, there is considerable genetic variation in the alleles that govern these pathways. Racial disparities across the life course are also complex factors that influence risk for all the diseases of late life (Whitfield and McClearn, 2005). Primary care providers operate on the front lines of this social minefield.

Effective, low-risk treatment for members of these diverse populations can be developed with a working knowledge of the underlying variation. Until these clinically relevant questions have been addressed through controlled clinical trials, genetics treatment technology will not be ready for routine use in the primary care of an aging population.

REFERENCES

Bernstein, A. B, E. Hing, A. J. Moss, et al. 2003. *Health Care in America: Trends in Utilization.* Hyattsville, MD: National Center for Health Statistics.

Caldwell, J. 2001. The pharmacogenetic basis of adverse drug reactions. *International Journal of Pharmaceutical Medicine* 15:83–84.

Canadian Task Force on Preventive Health Care. 2001. Colorectal cancer screening: Recommendation statement from the Canadian Task Force on Preventive Health Care. *Canadian Medical Association Journal* 165(2):206–8.

Ingelman-Sundberg, M. 2004. Genetic polymorphisms of cytochrome P450 2D6 (CYP2D6): Clinical consequences, evolutionary aspects, and functional diversity. *Pharmacogenomics Journal* 5:6–13.

Lindor, N. M., and M. H. Greene. 1998. The concise handbook of family cancer syndromes. Mayo Familial Cancer Program. *Journal of the National Cancer Institute* 90:1039–71.

Melzer D., A. Raven, D. E. Detmer, T. Ling, and R. L. Zimmern. 2003. *My Very Own Medicine: What Must I Know? Information Policy for Pharmacogenetics.* Cambridge, UK: University of Cambridge, Institute of Public Health, Department of Public Health and Primary Care.

Nelson, H. D., L. H. Huffman, R. Fu, and E. L. Harris. 2005. Genetic risk assessment and BRCA mutation testing for breast and ovarian cancer susceptibility: Systematic evidence review for the USPSTF. *Annals of Internal Medicine* 143: 362–79.

Palmer, L. I. 2003. Medical liability for pharmacogenomics. In *Pharmacogenomics: Social, Ethical and Clinical Dimensions,* ed. M. Rothstein. Pp. 187–206. Hoboken, NJ: Wiley-Liss.

Robbins, R., and S. Metcalfe. 2004. Integrating genetics as practices of primary care. *Social Science and Medicine* 59:223–33.

Shea, D. G., T. P. Miles, and M. Hayward. 1996. The health-wealth connection: Racial differences. *Gerontologist* 36(3):342–49.

Steimer, W., K. Zopf, S. von Amelunxen, H. Pfeiffer, J. Bachofer, J. Popp, et al. 2004. Allele-specific change of concentration and functional gene dose for prediction of steady-state serum concentrations of amitriptyline and nortriptyline in CYP2C19 and CYP2D6 extensive and intermediate metabolizers. *Clinical Chemistry* 50:1623–33.

Watson, E. K., D. Shickle, N. Qureshi, J. Emery, and J. Austoker. 1999. The new genetics and primary care: GPs' views on their role and their educational needs. *Family Practice* 16:420–25.

Whitfield, K. E., and G. McClearn. 2005. Genes, environment, and race. *American Psychologist* 60(1):104–14.

Winkelmann, B. R., J. Hager, W. E. Kraus, P. Merlini, et al. 2000. Genetics of coronary heart disease: Current knowledge and research principles. *American Heart Journal* 140(4):S11–12.

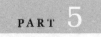

PART 5

ETHICAL AND
SOCIAL PERSPECTIVES

CHAPTER 16

Genetics, Aging, and Primary Care

Ethical Implications for Clinicians

PAMELA J. GRACE, PH.D.

The integration of new genetic knowledge into primary care practice provides an additional challenge for overburdened primary health
care clinicians, who already face a daily struggle to provide good basic care
to their patients in the face of financial, time, and other constraints. Yet a
major goal in both medicine and nursing, professions for which primary
care is a substantial area of practice, is to provide the sort of care that meets
the needs of patients. Both the medical and the nursing profession hold
their members morally accountable for providing effective services. Principle 1 of the American Medical Association Code of Medical Ethics asserts
that a "physician shall be dedicated to providing competent medical care,
with compassion and respect for human dignity and rights" (American
Medical Association, 2004–2005). Provision 3 of the American Nurses Association Code of Ethics for Nurses affirms that "the nurse promotes, advocates for, and strives to protect the health, safety, and rights of the patient" (American Nurses Association, 2001). While disciplinary codes of
ethics are formulated without the direct input of members of the public,

they are certainly predicated somewhat upon society's expectations of professionals (Grace, 1998).

Those who seek the services of primary care providers (PCPs) hope that they will receive appropriate assistance in evaluating risks, anticipating potential problems, and addressing current needs. For obvious reasons, the integration of current knowledge into practice is essential to the planning and delivery of care aimed at furthering patient good. Thus, among the responsibilities of PCPs is to understand the implications of genetic advances for their patient populations or, if the acquisition of such knowledge is beyond the provider's capacity, to be able to make referrals and direct patients toward appropriate resources.

Because the focus of this volume is the potential of genetic technology for addressing issues and problems associated with human aging, I use the following broad questions to frame my discussion: What are the responsibilities of primary care providers to gain genetic knowledge and to integrate it into their decision making, and what are the ethical implications of genetic testing for aging patients in primary care settings? However, it should be understood that genetic testing is only one of many ways of discovering a person's genetic risk factors.

Moral Responsibilities of the Primary Care Provider

Because primary health care is a service that provides for the patient's good by maintaining, protecting, or improving human functioning, primary care practice is an ethical or moral endeavor (Curtin and Flaherty, 1982; Pellegrino, 2001; Grace, 2002). I use the terms *ethical* and *moral* interchangeably in this context, although in everyday discourse they sometimes carry different meanings. The term *ethics* is "derived from the Greek ethos . . . meaning customs . . . conduct and character," and the term *moral* is derived from Latin *mores* and originally meant "to do with custom or habit" (Davis et al., 1997, 1). In health care settings, moral or ethical actions are those actions that are most likely to fulfill the purposes of the services sought or promised. Primary care providers thus can be criticized or praised to the extent that they strive to provide their patients with optimal care. By providing optimal care I mean undertaking the types of actions that are most likely to facilitate the person's well-being or comfort, given their current capacities and preexisting conditions.

Health care providers have a moral responsibility to use sound clinical judgment when applying genetic knowledge to the care of their patients in primary care settings and when eliciting information that may have genetic implications. This is because sound clinical judgments are those that are most likely to result in good actions or actions that will meet the goals of the decision-making process regardless of how, or by whom, the goals are formulated. Goals may be formulated by the provider with the patient's interests in mind, by the patient in response to provider questioning, by patients in collaboration with family members, or consensually. Sound clinical judgment requires that knowledge, skills, and experience are brought to bear on the issue at hand to formulate appropriate actions (Benner, Tanner, and Chesla, 1996; Downie and Macnaughton, 2000; Wulff and Gøtzsche, 2000). Clinical judgment takes into account the particular patient's context and other situational factors that are likely to facilitate or impinge on health. I understand that there are unresolved theoretical issues related to determining both the soundness of clinical judgments and which methods of decision making are most likely to yield good answers (Croskerry, 2000; Woll, 2002; Trede and Higgs, 2003; Paley, 2004). These issues cannot be adequately addressed here. However, most would agree that knowledge, skills, experience, and the motivation to provide for the patient's good are the minimal requirements for clinical judgments that consistently result in actions that are of benefit to the patient or to affected others. To this extent, we can say there is such a thing as sound clinical judgment.

Sound clinical judgment about the implications of genetic testing for patients necessarily takes into account the unique nature of a given patient's condition, values, and social context as well as any others who are likely to be affected. The knowledge base, besides what is required for primary care generally, will include at minimum a basic grasp of genetic concepts. The depth of understanding required will vary depending on the practice context and resources available. Resources that may be available (although they are generally in scarce supply) include genetic counselors, nurses with expertise or credentialing in genetics (International Society of Nurses in Genetics, 2005), or allied professionals with expertise in decision making related to the application of genetic advances. If such resources are not available, then the provider may need in-depth knowledge consistent with the needs of the patient population served.

Additionally, providers should have an understanding of the goals of genetic testing given the current state of the science and the characteristics of their particular practice population. When the practice population includes elderly patients, the goals of genetic testing may differ from those related to younger patients. The goals of genetic testing for younger people in primary care settings include ongoing surveillance for early detection of disease, prevention of disease by manipulating the patient's environment (e.g., diet and stress reduction in type 2 diabetes), or identifying heritable disease carriers for the purposes of family planning. However, when testing older patients who are symptomatic for genetically implicated diseases, the benefits may accrue to family members rather than to the patient in terms of screening or prevention. I argue later that under certain conditions patients may (with due consideration) be asked if they are willing to engage in genetic testing that has no direct benefit to them but that is likely to benefit others.

Finally, and perhaps most crucially, primary care providers have the responsibility to understand the limits of their knowledge, know where resources may be located, and consult with or make referrals to those schooled in ethical issues related to genetic testing such as the experts described above.

Genetics and Primary Care: Avoiding a Collision Course

Several authors have noted reluctance on the part of primary care providers to incorporate genetic knowledge into their primary care activities (Emery and Hayflick, 2001; Robins and Metcalfe, 2003; Burke, 2004; Van Riper and McKinnon, 2004). There are many reasons for this, including skepticism about the usefulness of incorporating such information into primary care practices, time constraints, and ignorance. However, increasingly our patients are forcing us to deal with the issue as they come to their appointments armed with questions stimulated by media advertising or news reports on innovations of interest to them. Our ethical responsibilities as clinicians will not allow us to ignore the subject of genetic advances. It is important that we actively undertake the pursuit of "genetic literacy" (Emery and Hayflick, 2001) so that we are able both to anticipate patients' needs for information and to interpret that information for them in a way that facilitates the achievement of their goals. There are many public misconceptions about what can be achieved by current genetic advances, and there are those who exploit this ignorance for economic gain

(Dalzell, 2001; Gray and Olopade, 2001; Hull and Prasad, 2001; Ratcliff, 2003).

Genetic Advances, Public Expectations, and Reality

Steve Jones (2000), a population geneticist, was commissioned by a group of health policy makers in the United States and the United Kingdom to formulate a report on genetic developments and their implications for health care delivery. In that report he points out the increasing public focus on developments in genetic knowledge. He postulates that one of the reasons for this is the alluring prospect that cures can be developed for many diseases. However, he cautions that while there have been worthwhile advances, there are also more limitations to the use of the new information than is commonly understood. The gap between public aspirations and current reality is already proving problematic for health care providers as they try to put new developments into perspective for their patients or try to avoid the issue altogether. In his opening statements, Jones (2000) comments that "most people die of a genetic disease but not many of them notice" (1). His point is that the functioning of genes is necessarily implicated in the aging process, in a multitude of diseases, in everyday living, and in obvious variations in human capacities. However, a host of other factors also influence both how well people are able to carry out daily activities and whether genetic mutations will result in disease. Genetic innovations on the near horizon are more likely to be helpful in diagnosing or predicting risk than in correcting disease (Jones, 2000). That is, we may be increasingly able to identify suspect genes or combinations of genes, but in most cases remedies for resulting symptoms or diseases have proven much more difficult to find. This is partly due to the complex interrelationships between genes, gene mutations, and environmental factors. On a more optimistic note, there are some promising developments related to predicting the metabolism of certain drugs based on genetic mutations, as discussed later. These developments are likely to benefit those requiring multiple pharmacological interventions as they will permit adjusting doses to more precisely match the patient's ability to metabolize the drug. This development, if effective, is likely to be of most benefit to elderly patients, as it is they who most frequently require multiple drugs for the treatment of chronic diseases.

Because many people do not understand the real scope and limits of genetic information, it is important that health care professionals, especially those in primary care settings, take seriously their obligation to assume responsibility for interpreting for patients and the public what is possible and under what circumstances. As Robins and Metcalfe (2003) note, "It is at the level of primary care that the prospect of genetic testing is first encountered" (223). Primary care providers also serve as a resource for unanswered questions related to media announcements of new drugs or new research. Indeed, there are currently many advertisements for drugs that tell the audience, "Ask your doctor if drug X or Y is right for you." Further, and where necessary, providers should be concerned to counter inaccurate claims made by those with commercial interests, such as direct-to-consumer marketers of genetic tests. Such tests carry the potential for harm that cannot necessarily be anticipated by the consumer. What is needed are skilled health care providers who can "guide [persons] through the complexities of genetic testing" and facilitate decisions about suitability for testing (Gray and Olopade, 2001, 3191). Thus, health care professionals need to develop a more sophisticated understanding of genetic advances than many currently possess. The reluctance on the part of many PCPs to incorporate genetic knowledge and information into the primary care skill set was noted earlier and is supported by research (Robins and Metcalfe, 2003). Nevertheless, we have a moral responsibility as providers to overcome this resistance and to pursue the knowledge needed for our individual practice.

Primary care providers need to understand the benefits and limits of applying genetic advances to the care of any patient, but perhaps especially to the care of their elderly patients, who might be supposed to have outlived, outwitted, or adapted to any inherent genetic disadvantages they possessed at birth. Providers' responsibilities include both understanding the scope and limits of their own knowledge related to genetics and continually updating this knowledge, using the demands of their particular practice as a guide to the sorts of knowledge necessary to meet their patients' needs. The application of genetic knowledge to the needs of elderly patients requires special consideration, as I will discuss shortly.

Gaining Genetic Knowledge: Understanding and Overcoming Resistance

While interest in, and knowledge of, genetic advances is becoming more common in a variety of specialty practices, Robins and Metcalfe (2003) point out that it is often in primary care settings where the issue of genetics and the genetic contributors to disease first arises. A report from the American Academy of Family Physicians (2004) points out that family physicians conduct 75 million more visits a year than providers in any other specialty. Further, family physicians are by no means the only providers of primary care. Others include nurse practitioners, physician's assistants, internists, and, in the case of aging patients, geriatricians. Because primary care providers are often the first health care professionals most patients encounter when seeking help with their health needs, it is in just such settings that practitioners need to be adequately prepared to assist their patients with decision making.

Emery and Hayflick (2001) argue that the most essential genetic skills for the primary care provider to master are assessing genetic risk via family history and communicating the implications of that risk. Yet PCPs are still not at that point. Robin and Metcalfe's (2003) qualitative study of Australian physicians, along with their review of the literature related to the incorporation of genetic knowledge into practice, highlights the fact that there is some ambivalence on the part of general practitioners toward integrating "genetics" into their practices. The resistance is not, to the extent that might be expected, related to becoming more genetically literate so much as to an "ontological problem of how genetics is to be located within the routines and practices" of their setting (Robin and Metcalfe, 2003, 225). Yet there is obvious pressure from various sources for PCPs to become more sophisticated in their genetic knowledge base.

There is a growing body of literature, from the disciplines of philosophy/ethics, medical history, nursing, and genetic counseling, concerned with various aspects of integrating knowledge and skills pertaining to genetics into primary care practice in order for providers to adequately address their patients' questions and needs. There is also an increased availability of genetics educational offerings specifically targeted to the practice needs of primary care providers. These educational endeavors are often geared toward encouraging partnerships between resources such as genetic counselors and the primary care provider. Part of the reason for this is that the most obvious or frequently asked question patients have is about the helpfulness of genetic testing for their particular situation or for their family members.

Primary Care Clinicians: Basic Skills in Genetics

A primary care genetics resource affirms, "The skills that GPs need to undertake work in genetics overlap with the skills that are used in everyday practice" (Oxford Primary Care Genetic Group, 2005). Burke (2004), recognizing that there are limits to the amount of time a primary care provider can spend with each patient, notes that the two most salient tasks for primary care providers are to learn "(a) how to identify patients who are candidates for a genetic workup—patients whose symptoms, physical findings, or family history suggest a genetic cause or risk; and (b) how to use genetic information most effectively to improve disease prevention" (1). Burke's article provides helpful strategies for time-pressed clinicians to facilitate genetic data-gathering. One of the main tools used to gather genetic information remains the family tree or pedigree. The Centers for Disease Control (2003) continue to advocate for the use of this in prevention. Several computerized tools are available, and some that will be especially useful in primary care are in the process of development. It is unclear, however, how helpful a family tree is for prevention of disease in elderly patients, for reasons suggested later. A family tree is more likely to assist the progeny of an elderly person than it is to assist the elderly person himself.

Effective completion of Burke's two important tasks requires that the primary care physician or nurse possess or acquire certain skills and characteristics. Integrating genetic advances into the project of facilitating primary health care will require (1) a basic knowledge of genetics; (2) an understanding of current developments—what can and cannot be accomplished; (3) the clinical sophistication that is a basic expectation for primary care practice, including the ability to ask hard questions about the goals of testing for particular patients or the usefulness of uncovering information; (4) a critical appraisal of each individual situation for the likely association between what Jones (2000) calls the "internal" (genetic) and "external" (environmental) causes of illness; and (5) the ability to effectively communicate information to patients, including the nature of the risks and benefits and for whom (in addition to the patient) the information gained might be beneficial or harmful.

Applications of Primary Care Genetic Skills to the Interests of Aging Patients

The knowledge and skills described above are perhaps especially important in the case of elderly patients. This is not to claim that elders are more vulnerable than younger people; they may be either more or less vulnerable than their younger counterparts. Rather, it is a reminder that in the data-gathering phase of the patient-practitioner meeting, the practitioner should be alert as usual to all possible contributors to the patient's current condition, including good health (in the case of an annual physical exam). Important considerations include asking what will be done with any genetically linked information that is uncovered in the history phase. It is critical to keep in mind the questions, Why test? and, What can be gained by verification? These are the ethical aspects of primary care decision making. That is, it is critical to discover what we need to know in order to promote a balance of good over bad consequences in clinical action.

Possible current and projected uses of genetic knowledge have been discussed in detail throughout this volume and include such innovations as repair of inborn genetic errors, identification of the likelihood of developing certain diseases, predictions of susceptibility to certain diseases, the ability to design drugs that are effective for the specific genetic makeup of certain patients (pharmacogonotics/pharmacogenomics), and applications for the purposes of treatment or symptom management.

A further important but relatively neglected area of study that perhaps relates more to people as they age than to younger people concerns the discovery of genetic factors that fortify someone against the development of disease. The results of this sort of research would inform health promotion and disease prevention strategies—an important focus of primary care.

Research is currently under way to identify suspect genes or patterns of genes in persons with "late-onset" maladies such as Alzheimer or Parkinson disease. Implicated gene mutations or polymorphisms have been uncovered for some forms of these diseases, and the hope is that cures for these diseases, or effective prevention strategies, might be discovered as a result of ongoing research. Thus, there may be an ethical justification for genetic testing in elderly patients who will not directly benefit from the testing, but the permissibility of such testing is dependent on the patient (or patient representative, in the case of cognitive impairment) giving informed consent. Guidelines for DNA diagnostic testing of patients with dementia symptoms are discussed more below. Generally, this sort of testing should be undertaken with extreme caution.

As noted earlier, testing for the presence of genes that predispose one to develop a certain disease is not likely to be a good reason to test older patients in primary care settings, for the simple reason that those patients have reached their current age despite any genetic predisposition. For aging persons, the most salient aspects of genetic advances are likely to be those that directly facilitate their personal health. For example, there is an increasing ability to use an individual's genetic information to prescribe drugs that are most efficient or most effectively metabolized by that person (pharmacogenomics). The U.S. Food and Drug Administration (FDA) approved the use of the AmpliChip CYP450 developed by the Roche pharmaceutical company (American Association of Retired Persons, 2005). This is a "Cytochrome P450 Genotyping Test, a DNA microarray used to analyze enzymes that play a role in metabolizing certain prescription drugs" (Young, 2005). It has the potential to permit the tailoring of drug dosages for a variety of drugs to an individual's metabolism, thus more precisely delivering the amount required for efficacy and minimizing side effects. Although approved for use by the FDA in December 2004, its efficacy in terms of accuracy, patient benefit, and cost effectiveness is not yet proven. Currently there is an identified gene mutation, HER–2, that results in a protein overexpression that is linked to breast cancer in some people who have the mutation. Identifying which breast cancer patients have this mutation permits personalized chemotherapy regimens (Young, 2005). It is likely that further discoveries of this sort will be made.

Genetic testing of elderly patients who exhibit symptoms of incurable diseases such as Alzheimer or Parkinson may yield information of interest to other family members or to future patients, in the event that a cure or prevention strategy is developed as a result of research, but it will not benefit the patient. However, genetic advances may also make such patients valuable sources of information for genetically related family members. Understanding how certain people avoid disease progression in spite of genetic susceptibility is an important focus of study. This avoids the mistake of focusing so heavily on a person's genetic makeup that realistic health promotion and health protection measures are neither suggested nor supported. Additionally, data about an individual's genetic risk factors are helpful for surveillance purposes, but to focus too narrowly on this misses the point that a person almost surely has unidentified genetic risk factors that are only indirectly hinted at by his or her health status or the health status of family members.

Because developments in genetics are occurring so rapidly, it will be difficult for primary care providers to stay current. However, PCPs are expected to keep up with other technological innovations such as new drugs, new laboratory tests, and new equipment, and as noted before there are increasing numbers of continuing-education offerings related to genetics. Additionally, a PCP can be well informed about genetic innovations but have problems applying this knowledge to the needs of patients. So an even more crucial aspect of the provider's responsibility is to understand the moral implications of genetic information related to their aging patients.

Ethical Issues, Genetic Testing, and Aging

The ethical responsibilities of primary care providers, as noted earlier, stem from the goals of primary care practice. To reiterate, those are generally understood to be promoting, maintaining, or protecting functioning or health and preventing disease. Patient visits necessarily focus on an exploration of a person's needs as related to these goals. For all patients there are potential risks as well as benefits to any data-gathering activity. For example, taking a detailed family history may reveal a pattern suggestive of a serious genetic variant and an associated risk of disease. Thus, the patient may receive disturbing information not anticipated from the nature of the visit. However, rather than detail all the ways in which harm can ensue from a seemingly simple primary care encounter, I will focus on the ethical implications of genetic testing in older people.

It might be helpful to look at a synthesis of commonly given reasons for genetic testing, given the current state of our knowledge. Genetic testing refers to a laboratory analysis of DNA or RNA from bodily tissues or fluids. Reasons for testing in the general population include the following:

1. Presymptomatic testing to identify people who may be at increased risk for contracting a disease because of a known gene mutation.

2. Diagnostic testing of a symptomatic individual whose symptoms suggest a genetic disorder.
3. Identification of a person's carrier status for the purposes of family planning.
4. Matching drug dosage with a person's ability to metabolize the drug.
5. Research that will lead to cures for disease, to the discovery of factors that delay onset of disease, or to improved prediction.

A primary care clinician would need to consider which of these constitutes a plausible consideration for an elderly patient given that patient's context, values, and preferences. Will presymptomatic testing provide useful information for the patient? It may if there are existing interventions or strategies that are likely to delay onset and if these interventions are not more onerous than the disease itself. However, this would be the patient's decision to make. The PCP's responsibility would be to facilitate the patient's autonomous choice. "Autonomous decision making requires an ability to process information and the freedom to make choices" (Grace and McLaughlin, 2005, 81). Thus, pertinent information about the risks and benefits of the testing should be shared with the patient in a process that allows the patient to make an informed decision. This requires a cognitively intact patient.

Several issues associated with presymptomatic genetic testing should be considered in the process of gathering information. There is the possibility of psychological harm from anticipating disease onset should the test be positive. A negative test result does not guarantee freedom from disease. The possibility of other unidentified gene mutations that increase the risk of disease is not ruled out. The familial nature of genetic information means that a positive finding has implications for other relatives. In fact, a positive finding may benefit a younger family member more than the elderly patient. Thus, the person being tested may be faced with the decision of whether to share the information gained. The patient may wish to be tested for the purpose of benefiting a family member; this is permissible if no coercion exists and other criteria for informed consent are met. The provider will need to ascertain whether there is any subtle or not so subtle pressure from other family members for the patient to get tested. Positive test results can put people at risk for loss of health insurance coverage or perhaps long-term care insurance. If the person is still working, he or she needs to consider whether information shared with employers will result in job loss. Although there are confidentiality protections in place for medical records, they are not airtight.

If the person is not capable of informed consent because of cognitive or other difficulties, then a proxy decision maker would need to make the decision on behalf of the patient. However, the decision should as closely as possible match what the individual would have wanted if capable of decision making. Thus, the substitute decision maker would be charged with providing a convincing defense of how the test would serve the patient's best interest based on knowledge of that person's lifestyle, values, and preferences.

It is possible that diagnostic DNA testing will eventually be available for many of the so-called late-onset disorders such as Alzheimer disease, Parkinson disease, and prostate cancer. As the American Geriatrics Society (2000) position statement notes, currently "the role of genetic testing for the prevention, diagnosis, and treatment of late onset disorders is uncertain." The statement cautions that such tests should not be routinely offered or ordered unless there is a clear idea of how they could benefit the patient and whether the results of the test might alter the care given.

It is possible that patients with early symptoms of dementing diseases such as Alzheimer's may wish to participate in research protocols that are designed to discover more about the disease. An elderly patient may be permitted to join such a research study for altruistic purposes—that is, because he or she wishes to contribute to the effort to find a cure. However, stringent safeguards are required to ensure that potential harm is minimized in the event that the subject is cognitively impaired or otherwise vulnerable. In such a case the primary care provider may be called on for advice. There are various resources delineating rules for research with human subjects. One good resource is available through the National Institutes of Health website (www.nihtraining.com/ohsrsite/info/sheet7.html).

The following brief discussion of ethical principles common in health care is offered as a further resource for primary care clinicians as they integrate knowledge of genetic advances into their practice. Several principles of ethics derived from a variety of moral theories can be relied upon to help direct practice or to clarify troubling issues. These principles have been explicated carefully by Beauchamp and Childress (2001), and I will give only a brief account here. While there are criticisms that these principles do not capture all of the problems that arise in health care settings and that sometimes they conflict with each other, offering no clear solutions, nevertheless they are heavily relied on for their ability to provide clarity in complex decision-making situations.

The principle of *autonomy* requires respect for an individual's right to make personal choices in health care. The exercise of autonomy requires that certain criteria are met. If the person is unable to process information properly (e.g., if cognitive or physical impairments impede judgment), or if he is unable to understand how various choices are likely to further or hinder his personal goals or whether the information obtained is inadequate or incomplete, then choices are unlikely to be autonomous (Beauchamp and Childress, 2001). As described earlier, autonomy is the principle that underlies ideas of informed consent. Although it can be argued that the principle of autonomy represents an ideal, in that we are all subject to internal and external influences on our action, in general people are deemed to have the right of self-determined choices if they can meet the above criteria.

The principle of *nonmaleficence* requires that we do no harm, or that any harm that does accrue to a patient in the course of treatment is outweighed by the likely benefit.

Beneficence is represented by the goals of health care in general, and primary health care in particular. It is the health care provider's responsibility to further the patient's good, given professional standards and the goals of care.

Justice in health care is generally viewed as the fair distribution of the benefits and burdens inherent in promoting the health of society. Among the implications of justice in primary health care is the idea that people, including elderly persons, be allowed to participate in research that is likely to benefit either them or a future cohort of like patients.

Respect for a patient's autonomy has gained strength over the last few decades and is a prevalent consideration in all clinical settings in the United States. Respecting autonomy also generally means respecting the patient's privacy and keeping his or her information confidential. This respect for patient autonomy is an expectation of the patient/provider relationship, which is best described as fiduciary in nature. That is, the patient lacking information or the wherewithal to meet his or her own health care needs is forced to trust that the provider will keep both the patient's best interests in mind when assessing needs and planning interventions and will support the patient's autonomous choice in providing adequate infor-

mation to support this. However, the familial nature of any genetic knowl
edge gained about an individual complicates this emphasis on autonomy, because the information gained carries the potential to affect or even harm another family member, and harm to others has generally been seen as a brake or limit on the power of patient autonomy. Respecting patient autonomy in the context of gathering genetic information requires providers to have conversations with their patients about the implications of their personal data for kin. Relatives of the patient may well also be patients in your care, and this can create a conflict of interest if the information gained about one patient has implications for the other patient's health.

Family elders may hold the keys to family secrets. Some families have unwritten rules that forbid discussion of patterns of illnesses within the family. Thus, it may be difficult to get a good family history or develop a family pedigree for other family members within the particular primary care practice. Clinical judgment should be used in deciding how to approach the patient about sharing this information when it might make a difference to the care or testing recommendations for other family members. Finally, those elderly people who have diseases with a genetic component but have survived might provide clues that permit appropriate health-promoting endeavors for others.

Conclusion

Primary care providers have responsibilities incurred by their member ship in a health care profession and as outlined in their standards of practice and code of ethics. The professional responsibilities for providing a "good" or service for society and its members include accountability for remaining knowledgeable, skilled, and capable of interpreting the advantages and disadvantages of new technologies so that their usefulness for the particular patient population is known. There are special considerations related to incorporating genetic innovations into primary care practice with older persons. The current status of genetic testing is such that it should be undertaken in elderly persons only with that person's informed consent and after due consideration of the possible benefits and harms to the person.

REFERENCES

American Academy of Family Physicians. 2004. *Position Statement: Issues of Genetic Health.* www.aafp.org/x24762.xml.

American Association of Retired Persons. 2005. *Bulletin Board: The Right Drugs for Your DNA.* Washington, DC: AARP.

American Geriatrics Society. 2000. *Position Statement: Genetic Testing for Late-onset Alzheimer's Disease.* www.americangeriatrics.org/staging/positionpapers/gen_testPF.shtml.

American Medical Association. 2004–2005. *Code of Medical Ethics: Current Opinions with Annotations.* Chicago: AMA Press.

American Nurses Association. 2001. *Code of Ethics for Nurses with Interpretive Statements.* Washington, DC: ANA.

Beauchamp, T. L., and J. F. Childress. 2001. *Principles of Biomedical Ethics,* 5th ed. New York: Oxford University Press.

Benner, P., C. A. Tanner, and C. A. Chesla. 1996. *Expertise in Nursing Practice: Caring Clinical Judgment and Ethics.* New York: Springer.

Burke, W. 2004. Genetic testing in primary care. *Annual Review of Genomics and Human Genetics* 5:1–14.

Centers for Disease Control and Prevention, Office of Genomics and Disease Prevention. 2003. *Genomics and Population Health: United States.* Atlanta, GA: CDC. www.cdc.gov/genomics/activities/ogdp/2003.htm.

Croskerry, P. 2000. The cognitive imperative: Thinking about how we think. *Academic Emergency Medicine* 7:1223–31.

Curtin, L., and M. J. Flaherty. 1982. *Nursing Ethics: Theories and Pragmatics.* Bowie, MD: Brady Communications, Prentice-Hall.

Dalzell, M. D. 2001. Genetic medicine: Powerful opportunities for good and greed. *Managed Care* 5. www.managedcaremag.com/archives/0105/0105.genetics.html.

Davis, A., M. A. Aroskar, J. Liaschenko, and T. S. Drought. 1997. *Ethical Dilemmas and Nursing Practice,* 4th ed. Stamford, CT: Appleton and Lange.

Downie, R. S., and J. Macnaughton. 2000. *Clinical Judgment: Evidence in Practice.* New York: Oxford University Press.

Emery, J., and S. Hayflick. 2001. The challenge of integrating genetic medicine into primary care. *British Journal of Medicine* 322:1027–30.

Grace, P. J. 1998. *A Philosophical Analysis of the Concept of Advocacy: Implications for Provider-Patient Relationships.* University of Tennessee. UMI Proquest. Digital Dissertations. AAT 9923287.

Grace, P. J. 2002. Philosophies, models, and theories: Moral obligations. In *Nursing Theory: Utilization and Application,* 2nd ed., ed. M. R. Alligood and A. Marriner-Tomey. Pp. 63–79. St. Louis: Elsevier/Mosby.

Grace, P. J., and M. McLaughlin. 2005. Ethics column: When consent isn't informed enough. *American Journal of Nursing* 105(4):79–85.

Gray, S., and O. I. Olopade. 2001. Editorial: Direct-to-consumer marketing of genetic tests for cancer: Buyer beware. *Journal of Clinical Oncology* 21:3191–93.

Hull, S. C., and K. Prasad. 2001. Reading between the lines: Direct-to-consumer advertising of genetic testing in the USA. *Reproductive Health Matters* 9(18): 44–48.

International Society for Nurses in Genetics. 2005. *Academic Programs.* www.isong .org/.

Jones, S. 2000. *Genetics in Medicine: Real Promises, Unreal expectations.* New York: Milbank Memorial Fund.

Oxford Primary Care Genetic Group. 2005. *Topics in Primary Care: GP Skills.* www. dphpc.ox.ac.uk/opcgg/topics.htm#1.

Paley, J. 2004. Clinical cognition and embodiment. *International Journal of Nursing Studies* 41:1–13.

Pellegrino, E. D. 2001. The internal morality of clinical medicine: A paradigm for the ethics of the helping and healing professions. *Journal of Medicine and Philosophy* 26:559–79.

Ratcliff, N. 2003. Marketing genetics: The need for consumer protection. *Consumer Policy Review* 13(1):8–15.

Robins, R., and S. Metcalfe. 2003. Integrating genetics as practices of primary care. *Social Science and Medicine* 59:223–33.

Trede, F., and J. Higgs. 2003. Re-framing the clinician's role in collaborative clinical decision making: Re-thinking practice knowledge and the notion of clinician-patient relationships. *Learning in Health and Social Care* 2(2):66–73.

Van Riper, M., and W McKinnon. 2004. Genetic testing for breast and ovarian cancer susceptibility: A family experience. *Journal of Midwifery and Women's Health* 49(3):210–19.

Woll, S. 2002. *Everyday Thinking. Memory, Reasoning, and Judgment in the Real World.* Mahwah, NJ: Lawrence Erlbaum Associates.

Wulff, H. R., and P C Gøtzsche. 2000. *Rational Diagnosis and Treatment: Evidence Based Clinical Decision Making,* 3rd ed. Malden, MA: Blackwell Science.

Young, D. 2005. Scientists focus on pharmacogonomics at FDA science forum. *American Journal of Health System Pharmacy* 62:1226.

Aging, Genetics, and Social Justice

LISA SOWLE CAHILL, PH.D., AND
SARAH MOSES, PH.D.(C)

The rapid emergence and marketing of new genetic technologies press upon us urgent questions about the roles of medicine and science in modern societies. Technologies to alleviate or even arrest the aging process are no exception. A particularly difficult question concerns the impact of genetic discoveries on society, comprised of all who have a need for and a claim on its resources. This chapter will make the case that antiaging technologies are likely to be marketed to elites in prosperous societies, with at least two dangerous consequences for the common good. First, the aging process will be medicalized in a way that actually impedes access to and enjoyment of the authentic conditions of a worthwhile life in old age, even for those who can afford the new interventions. Second, a highly technological approach to the achievement of a "good" aging process will funnel resources away from universal access to basic health care and other services, for elderly and nonelderly people alike, in the United States and abroad.

Placing genetic technologies within the larger framework of social justice and participation helps resolve whether or not these technologies are likely to enhance the experience of old age and whether they promote or undermine solidarity in the common good. This framework places genetic research within a larger perspective on the various forms of support for elderly persons and on the contributions elderly persons may make to others.

The approach to be adopted here is indebted to the social tradition of Catholicism (see O'Brien and Shannon, 1992; Hollenbach, 2002). We believe that the basic framework and values this tradition advances will be amenable to all those interested in social justice in health care. A central premise of this tradition is that the common good of society is more than the good of its more powerful members, and even more than the individual goods of all members taken in the aggregate. The common good, ideally and normatively understood, mandates the solidarity of all in social structures and processes that enable everyone to share cooperatively in the basic political and material goods of society. The common good includes the practices and institutions through which solidarity and mutual rights and duties are expressed and enabled, and that create and mediate the goods a society provides.

Participation in these practices and institutions, interdependently with other members of the social body, is itself a key component of a share in the common good. The ability to actively fulfill one's own capabilities and aspirations while helping others to do the same is as essential to enjoyment of the common good as is the derivation of personal goods and benefits. A statement by the U.S. Catholic Bishops captures the importance of the concept of participation for measuring justice in a society: "Basic justice demands the establishment of minimum levels of participation in the life of the human community. The ultimate injustice is for a person or group to be treated actively or abandoned passively as if they were nonmembers of the human race. To treat people this way is effectively to say they simply do not count as human beings" (U.S. Catholic Bishops, 1986, §77). The common good, so understood, is achieved through cooperation within and among individuals, families, and local communities as well as through solidarity with more distant persons and social groups. Understood in the context of elderly people, a U.N. document explained the principle of participation in this way: "Older persons should remain integrated in society, participate actively in the formulation and implementation of policies that directly affect their well-being and share their knowledge and skills with younger generations" (United Nations, 1999).

This framework will shape our consideration of genetic technology and elderly people. After discussing the situations of elderly persons in contemporary culture and medicine, we will focus on the key ethical question of participation of elderly people in the common good, comprehensively understood. Catholic social categories will be employed to delineate the importance of participation for elderly people. Furthermore, a consideration of the Community of Sant'Egidio and its work with elderly people will serve as a concrete illustration of the basic goods needed to assure this participation.

Elderly Persons in Contemporary Culture and Medicine

Richard Sprott opens the door to these issues in chapter 1 of this book with the apt title, "Reality Check: What Is Genetic Research on Aging Likely to Produce, and What Are the Ethical and Clinical Implications of Those Advances?" Sprott does not predict that "we are going to see 150-year-old humans anytime soon," but he is confident that "we will find new, effective therapies for age-related diseases." For example, designer drugs keyed to one's genetic makeup will be both more effective and better able to avoid deleterious side effects. It may be possible even to replace defective genes with healthy ones or to provide the products that malfunctioning genes should be producing. Research on telomeres, the DNA that determines the lifespan of cells, is a particularly promising type of investigation into the aging process and the diseases that most frequently accompany aging, such as cancer. Such research holds the potential to improve quality of health in old age, which is certainly a laudable goal. This chapter aims to evaluate the research directions and therapeutic possibilities identified by Sprott in several contexts: the value and role of elderly people in the perspective of society; the variety of factors that make up a satisfying and secure old age; and a variety of other demands on social resources.

In the United States, at least three-quarters of people reach old age before they die. Death usually occurs in hospitals and, to a lesser extent, in nursing homes (Institute of Medicine, 1997). Government statistics predict that by 2040, the average 65-year-old American will live to age 85, six and a half years longer than in 1940 (Diamond and Orszag, 2005). Modern medicine has all but eliminated early death from infectious diseases like malaria and tuberculosis, at least for those fortunate enough to reside in the economically privileged areas of the globe. In developed nations, the leading causes of death in old age are heart disease, cancer, and stroke (Institute of Medicine, 1997).

In prosperous societies, elderly people enter into their "golden years" in better health and with greater capacity to enjoy new interests and activities. Yet a diminishing of physical and mental abilities is an inevitable part of the aging process. As longevity increases, so does the likelihood that life will end in a prolonged period of decline due to the diseases that are related to later life (President's Council on Bioethics, 2005, 1–11). Yet decline and death are increasingly seen as "outside the norm." They are neither well tolerated nor integrated as part of the anticipated life process.

Our purpose here is not to oppose extending the average length of life within reasonable limits or improving health in the final third of life. In fact, access to better basic health care and other technology has already increased length of life in the past century. And length of life will likely increase further, with or without genetic research. Sprott is certainly right that, even if the lifespan does not expand to 150 years, it would be beneficial to "find new, effective therapies for age-related diseases." However, the critical ethical issue is just resource allocation that represents solidarity in the common good for both elderly and nonelderly people and for all economic groups. Sprott concludes rightly that the problem of just or discriminatory resource allocation is "*the* central ethical question" behind the development of antiaging technologies.

The Principle of Participation

While genetic research holds promise for improving health in later life, elderly people require more than high-tech medicine. The principle of participation demands that we place resource allocation for genetic research within the larger context of the family and community assistance and basic care needed to maximize social participation, to cope with losses, and to adjust goals to remaining strengths in one's final years.

A pervasive cultural ethos of individual independence and market exchange makes those who seem socially unproductive, or who require assistance with basic, daily tasks of self-care, seem like a burden to themselves and those around them. To the extent that genetic advances can decrease disease and disability in late life, they also could facilitate greater participation in society by elderly people, by allowing people, for example, to live at home longer with better health and even to extend their working years. In the meantime, it is important not to let the immediate and concrete needs of elderly people be overshadowed by research that promises eventual benefits primarily for the generation now funding and carrying out the research. Ethically, we need to remain focused on the elderly people of today and the larger question of how our society can support the greater number of people living to and in old age, especially because disease and disability will never be completely eradicated.

A 2002 background paper on aging research, prepared for the President's Council on Bioethics, found that current medical investigation is going beyond the diseases of elderly people (e.g., Parkinson, Alzheimer, and cardiovascular diseases). It concurred with Sprott that research is proliferating in areas like the lengthening of the lifespan and the prevention of deterioration in old age in general. Specific research topics include free radicals and mitochondrial dysfunction, caloric restriction, the genetics of aging, regenerative medicine, and hormone treatments to slow aging (President's Council on Bioethics, 2002). This background paper raised ethical questions on the likely effects of projected discoveries on the populations with the resources to use them. "How could our ability to control the length of life affect our thinking about the breadth and depth of life? . . . How will social and political institutions—like the education system, the retirement system, the health care and insurance systems—deal with such changes?" (2–3). Most of the world's people will have difficulty accessing such "remedies" for old age.

Even in the United States, there is no guarantee that health insurers would support major, expensive expansion of coverage. In addition, there are more than 47 million people with no insurance at all. The U.S. political climate resists continued or expanded funding of programs that benefit elderly citizens, especially Social Security and Medicaid. In turn, this raises concern that genetic technologies that could benefit elderly people are not likely to become widely available. As the large postwar "boomer" generation ages, a smaller workforce worries about protecting its own assets more than about carrying an economic load for the older generation. In the words of Catholic political commentator E. J. Dionne, "The retired millionaire playing golf in Palm Springs is spoken of as if he is in the same class as the elderly widow in a modest apartment in Cleveland . . . Most seniors who use Medicare and rely on Social Security desperately need the help to stay out of poverty" (Dionne, 2005, 9). The recent debate about the future of the U.S. government–funded Social Security program, instituted in 1935, after the Great Depression, to protect all American workers in their old age, suggests that protection of elderly people is growing increasingly precarious. In fact, for 20 percent of the elderly people in this country, Social Security is their exclusive source of income (Dionne, 2005).

Medicaid funding is another area of concern affecting elderly people. Unlike Social Security, from which all workers benefit in retirement, Medicaid is a means-tested program, created to provide medical care for the poor. It provides care for more than 52 million people of all ages. To be eligible, applicants must have no more than $2,000, though they may continue to own homes, a provision that is now being contested by critics who want to limit eligibility. The federal government and the states share the cost of Medicaid, with the federal contribution ranging among states from 50 percent to 77 percent.

Though a means-tested program, Medicaid is used by many elderly people. In a typical scenario, an elderly middle-class woman uses up her resources caring for her husband and needs nursing care herself. Medicaid pays for about two-thirds of the nation's 1.6 million nursing home residents. About half of all people over 85 are in nursing homes. The increased chance of institutionalization after the age of 85 has significant implications when one considers that this population is expected to grow from the current size of 4 million to 19 million people by 2050 (Federal Interagency Forum on Aging-Related Statistics, 2000, 2). Medicaid takes 22 percent of the average state budget, more than is spent on elementary and secondary education. Because the burden of Medicaid on states is so great, state governors are calling for an overhaul of the program (Harris, 2005). The situation of Medicaid illustrates several important points: many people lack adequate resources to care for themselves in old age; government programs are necessary to supplement the presently scant health care resources of many elderly persons; and social trends favor contraction rather than expansion of public support for essential needs of elderly people.

Disadvantaged racial and ethnic groups obviously have greater rates of poverty and have less access to social services in general. This fact has a disproportionate effect on elderly people, and on women within the elderly population.[1] Because women live, on average, a few years longer than men, there are more elderly women than men requiring care and support. Poverty results not only in exclusion from direct health resources, including both preventive and acute care, but also in poor housing, poor nutrition, less education, and fewer means of access to available supports, including supports for the caregivers in one's family or network, who are typically also women.

Elderly people and their caregivers often have limited access to social and economic resources, a key source of stress and isolation. In modern societies the privatization and mobility of the nuclear family, as well as divorce, mean that caregivers are often cut off from networks of family and friends who share responsibilities and provide relief. A solidaristic and community-oriented appreciation of justice for elderly people will identify an obligation of society and government to create and subsidize structures that enhance family and neighborhood care. From the perspective of social justice, there is also a social obligation to ensure income security, health care, and housing arrangements that facilitate the continued participation of elderly people in community activities and goals, to the best extent possible for each individual.

Social Justice, Genetics, and Aging

Social justice concerns are not pertinent only to genetics or only to aging. Yet justice questions become strikingly acute when genetics is applied to aging, for at least three reasons. First, genetics is a quickly developing area of investment for a profit-driven pharmaceutical industry, and the baby-boomers have been and continue to be a major target market. Within this population, the small proportion of the very rich outweighs, from a marketing standpoint, the majority with modest incomes and limited health insurance. The medicalization of old age creates a dynamic in the economics of health care in which new technologies are financed by rising insurance premiums, putting a greater burden on the young and healthy, taking away resources from long-term care, and driving more people out of the insurance pool (Ter Meulen, 2002).

Second, elderly people in general are already a population that is often unable to access social resources of a variety of types, health related and otherwise.

Third, many needs of elderly people are more urgent than gene therapy, like housing, basic health care, transportation, and assistance with household tasks. Elderly people often lack networks that not only provide care but also enable their continued contributions to and participation in society. Because such problems are immediate and their potential solutions relatively clear, while gene therapy is hypothetical and prospective, a social justice perspective demands that such needs not be compromised by resource allocation directed toward genetic technology.

In fact, there are good examples of organizations trying to meet the fundamental, basic needs of elderly people, and we offer their work as illustrative of the areas that need to be a priority in resource allocation. While genetic technology related to aging is rightly focused on the future goal of lessening disease and disability related to old age, a larger ethical vision rooted in social justice challenges society also to use resources for elderly people today and for the *immediate* basic needs that we know exist now. More effective ways to address the needs of elderly people are everyone's responsibility and are possible at many levels.

One example is the Catholic Health Association, a professional organization for Roman Catholic health care facilities, health care systems, community clinics, nursing and rehabilitation facilities, and so on. The CHA has a long track record of enabling cooperation among health facilities, social services, and networks of community care for elderly people and their families. Its website includes information and advocacy opportunities for members.[2] Special priorities are enhancing care across the life continuum, serving vulnerable populations, and advocating for expanded health insurance and government programs serving sick, elderly, and poor people.

A less well known example, though with international scope, is the Community of Sant'Egidio, which especially prioritizes opportunities for social participation even for those elderly people who experience late-life disease and disability. The Community of Sant'Egidio is a lay volunteer organization that began in Rome in 1968 but today is present in many countries, including the United States. While its roots are in the Roman Catholic Church, Sant'Egidio is ecumenical in its membership and is known for its participation in interreligious dialogue and partnership. Sant'Egidio began working with elderly people in 1972, and, echoing our earlier discussion of the concept of participation, it articulates the fundamental need and desire of elderly people in this way: "Indeed, the elderly ask a question of integration, of company, that is not only a demand for solidarity and social services. It is a question of full participation in social life."[3] Thus, Sant'Egidio seeks to foster the participation of older people through basic care at home, providing health care, intergenerational friendship, and partnership in various volunteer initiatives.[4]

One of the main ways that Sant'Egidio serves the participation of elderly people is through its efforts to enable them to remain at home. Given the realities of today's contemporary society, many elderly people are unable to enjoy the assistance of strong, local family networks. Even when an elderly person has family assistance, it may be difficult to access all of the help needed. Many elderly people are forced into institutional settings, not because of real medical need but because they lack assistance with basic daily tasks or with the financial means to access such home services. Sant'Egidio's members voluntarily provide weekly, sometimes daily, visitation to elderly people living at home, provide transportation and accompaniment for doctor's appointments, and administer or coordinate medications.

Sant'Egidio also assists elderly people in accessing government and private services. Sant'Egidio groups work in their local contexts with government and other private agencies that provide elder services in order to maximize the possibility for elderly people to remain participants in their community. One of the best examples of these local coordinating efforts is a book published by Sant'Egidio organizations in their local city called *How to Remain in Your Own Home When You Are Elderly*. This easily understood publication coordinates information such as health centers and doctors, cultural and activity centers, governmental and nonprofit agencies, and transportation options. Thus, while providing a great deal of basic care and assistance to elderly people themselves, Sant'Egidio groups also use the health care and social services structures already in place in a local area. In fact, Sant'Egidio groups are often able to develop long-term personal associations with local agencies and elder care workers, including housekeeping and financial management services.

The experience of Sant'Egidio illustrates that for elderly people to enjoy their late life as a time of purpose and participation, more is required than high-tech medicine; it involves the provision and coordination of basic home and health services combined with reliable relationships in their community and family. Especially for low- and middle-income elderly people, such services must remain a priority in any discussion of resource allocation directed toward elderly people, especially toward the medical and nonmedical services *available now* that can help to maintain participation even with the limitations of late-life disease and disability.

The work of Sant'Egidio and the experience of old age is illustrated by the story of Mary, an 86-year-old unmarried elderly woman living in a major U.S. city. Mary emigrated to the United States as a young woman and has no other family in the country. She lives alone in a one-bedroom apartment in a public housing development. Mary enjoys fairly good health, needing only two different prescription pills per day for manageable conditions. However, friends recently found her collapsed on the floor of her apartment with a slight sprain to her ankle. After evaluation at the hospital, doctors determined that Mary's collapse had been due to nutritional imbalance and dehydration.

After a short stay at the hospital, doctors were planning to place Mary in a nursing home because they felt it was still unsafe for her to be at home alone. However, members of Sant'Egidio were able to work out an alternative plan, relying on the relationship they had established with her doctor. The volunteers set up a short-term rotating schedule, taking turns staying at Mary's apartment overnight, so as to avoid the need for a stay in a nursing home, and facilitated her recovery to independent living. The volunteers assisted with her medicine regimen, provided for greater independence by acquiring an automated pill dispenser, cooked meals, and made sure that Mary was drinking enough fluids.

They also coordinated local elder services to put together resources that Mary now needed on a permanent basis, such as home health and hygiene assistance and twice-weekly attendance at a senior center affiliated with a nearby hospital, which offered therapeutic exercise and activities.[5] The group also arranged for a "money manager" to pay bills and keep track of finances. Sant'Egidio continues to involve Mary in various activities of the local Sant'Egidio group in her apartment building, including visiting other elderly people at a nearby nursing home.

Mary's story illustrates that creativity and a few resources can place elderly people in networks of services that encourage continuing social participation in old age and facilitate the connections with community and the larger society so essential to a worthwhile life. However, it should be noted that many of the services arranged for Mary are funded by state and federal resources that are affected by public policy decisions regarding resource allocation. While genetic technologies may someday enable people like Mary to postpone or escape a decline in capabilities, it can hardly be overemphasized that funding for research on such technologies can be only a part—and perhaps a small part—of an ethical social approach to aging. Although Sant'Egidio and the Catholic Health Association are inspired by religious ideals, their concern for vulnerable elderly people and their ability to improve the daily and immediate situation of elders *should not be limited to* churches, synagogues, mosques, and other faith communities. A just society that invests in all its members will work hard to ensure that those facing old age will do so with the support of their families, communities, and government.

The importance of basic services and care becomes clear if one looks at a study of those seeking physician-assisted suicide in the state of Oregon. From the perspective of actual patients, the study examines the most important needs and anxieties of those facing the inevitable and steady diminishment of capacities. Data collected on those who chose to end their lives underline what is necessary to make life in decline worthwhile. Only 22 percent gave pain as a reason for their decision, 33 percent feared becoming a burden to family members, and 2 percent mentioned financial constraints. (Of course, financial resources would also make it possible for elderly people to avoid becoming a burden to family, or in other words to be cared for by family members who have adequate support in carrying out the responsibility.) Prevalent in the determination that life was no longer worthwhile was a feeling that autonomy and independence had been lost (85%), "decreased ability to participate in enjoyed activities" (79%), and loss of control over bodily functions (58%).[6]

Genetic approaches to aging could certainly help alleviate some of these problems, by slowing down mental decline and loss of physical function, control, and mobility. However, it is questionable whether these outcomes could be avoided entirely, especially in view of lengthened years of life, in which the decline would simply be postponed (and perhaps prolonged) rather than eliminated. Moreover, the Oregon survey found that a large majority (79%) of those seeking physician-assisted suicide had cancer, one disease that new medical options have not been able to decrease among elderly people. The Oregon statistics certainly recommend a longer and deeper look at the genuine needs that accompany the aging process, especially as it involves disability and disease. A comprehensive approach would integrate the biologically based components and determinants of aging with psychosocial determinants and would rely on long-term care and social and relational remedies for the deficits of aging, at least as much as on medical genetics.

Conclusion

If genetic technologies can contribute to better health in later life and thus facilitate ongoing participation by elderly persons, then social justice also asks, What measures are needed to ensure that all elderly people enjoy just access to these benefits? Who will pay for the genetic technologies that roll back the pace of aging, and who will get to use them? Will the population that does not have more fundamental needs met be the same one that gets, say, replacement genes, or will it be the population on the golf course in Palm Springs? Without proper government intervention through regulation and funding, allocation decisions will be made by drug manufacturers that determine which disease or disability is most likely to bring in a profit (Angell, 2004). The people in this country who will be least likely to receive gene therapies for aging will be women (who are poor in old age more often than men), African Americans, Native Americans, many Hispanics, recent immigrants, and of course all those with inadequate health insurance. Given the United Nations' demographic projections for the reality of aging societies in the developing world, there is a compelling ethical question concerning global access to these technologies (United Nations, 2003). The issues of economic disparity and just access were captured in a statement by a U.N. official concerning the reality of aging in the developing world: "In Europe, countries got rich before they became old. But in the developed world, countries are growing old before they are rich" (New York Times, 2002).

More than a decade ago, a joint report on social justice for elderly people was produced by the Hastings Center (a pioneering U.S. bioethics institute) and a Dutch counterpart. The report concluded that health care should be viewed in light of larger public policy concerns, values, and priorities, to produce a holistic approach to quality of life during the aging process. Solidarity between the generations should be nurtured, as the basis for a just and workable system, accommodating the contributions and needs of all (Joint International Research Group, 1994). According to the study, old age should not be made into a medical problem but should be viewed as the corollary to youth. Childhood and old age should be provided for in tandem, expressing the commitment and investment of the whole society. The burden of caregiving on women should be alleviated through more informal sharing and government support programs. It was recommended that elders themselves organize politically and collectively, not to avoid their own responsibilities for child-directed goods such as education but to advocate that health and welfare be united in comprehensive programs. The public dialogue on the significance of old age should be advanced at all levels of society through the media, education, and joint public-private initiatives.

Precisely this type of dialogue was promoted by the United Nations when it declared 1999 the Year of the Older Person, with the theme "a society for all ages."[7] Many different organizations and agencies were invited to consider how a truly intergenerational society could be built, wherein "every individual, each with rights and responsibilities, has an active role to play." Subsequently, the United Nations published a document called the *United Nations Principles for Older Persons* to assure that "priority attention" would be given to the needs and aspirations of elderly people (United Nations, 1999). This document encouraged governments to incorporate into their national programs these five principles for older people: independence, participation, care, self-fulfillment, and dignity.

An example of such national dialogue is a working paper for the U.S. Department of Housing and Urban Development, which similarly recommended legislation that could lead in this country to "a national health and housing policy agenda" that ensures access to subsidized housing for elderly people and a coordinated continuum of other kinds of care. These would include support services, social services, and health care. Such services would permit all those in the aging process to maintain relative independence and social connections as long as possible (Elderly Housing Coalition Committee on the Continuum of Care, 2000). Such a housing policy is in line with the principle of independence, which was articulated by the United Nations as including the goal, "Older persons should be able to reside at home for as long as possible" (United Nations, 1999).

In the words of two commentators writing from the vantage point of Catholic social teaching, "Although new patterns of aging create new troubles for families and community, they create new opportunities" (Cochran and Cochran, 2003, 94). All persons have reciprocal responsibilities and rights within the common good, and our discussion of the work of the Community of Sant'Egidio illustrated the way in which one organization attempts to facilitate the participation and contribution of elderly people.

Solidarity in the common good underwrites a compassionate, creative, and proactive approach to the fact that the needs of everyone vary throughout the lifespan. No one is immune to the contingencies of health status, income, and socioeconomic class: "Human social dependence is not an evil to be overcome ('I don't want to be a burden on my children') but instead a facet of the richness of community living . . . Moreover, because humans are social creatures, it is natural and good that society share the burdens of both childhood and old age" (Cochran and Cochran, 2003, 94).

The purpose of this chapter has been to argue that social justice demands that we take seriously all the forces that result in pushing elderly people to the margins of society and thus deny their participation in the common good. Genetic therapies aimed at improving health by correcting late-life disease and disability can contribute to the participation of elderly people by removing the health-related barriers to participation. However, there are also factors involving basic personal care, assistance in the daily task of living, and human connections in the community that must not be neglected in resource allocation for elderly people.

NOTES

1. For further discussion of the particular vulnerability of elderly women, see Williamson (1997)

2. The CHA website is www.chausa.org.

3. Information on the Community of Sant'Egidio's work with elderly people can be accessed at www.santegidio.org/en/soliderieta/anziani/index.htm.

4. While Sant'Egidio is an example of an organization pursuing these goals from a Christian perspective, such practices and philosophy are certainly not exclusive to the Christian tradition. For example, Jewish agencies in Boston under Combined Jewish Philanthropies initiated a program to provide supportive home services with the aim of enabling elders to retain the independence of living at home and to continue participating in their communities (see www.cjp.org). For further discussion of multicultural and multifaith responses to aging, see Cahill and Mieth (1991), Hermalin (2002), and Makoni and Stroeken (2002).

5. As a low-income senior, Mary would be unable to afford the homemaker services and attend the senior center without a subsidy that she receives through the city's elder services office—a clear example of the kind of basic services that must remain a priority for spending aimed at elderly people.

6. Statistics are available on the Oregon Health Division website (www.ohd .hr.state.or.us/shc/pas/an-index.htm) and from the advocacy organization Com-

passion in Dying (info@compassionindying.org). These statistics were taken from a Compassion in Dying brochure, "Compassion in Dying Federation."

7. Information can be accessed at www.un.org/esa/socdev/ageing/ageing/ageall .htm.

REFERENCES

Angell, M. 2005. *The Truth about the Drug Companies: How They Deceive Us and What to Do about It.* New York: Random House.

Cahill, L. S., and D. Mieth, eds. 1991. *Aging.* Philadelphia: Trinity Press International.

Cochran, C. E., and D. C. Cochran. 2003. *Catholics, Politics, and Public Policy: Beyond Left and Right.* Maryknoll, NY: Orbis Books.

Diamond, P. A., and P. Orszag. 2005. Saving Social Security: A balanced approach. Cited in Robin Toner and David E. Rosenbaum. In overhaul of Social Security, age is the elephant in the room. *New York Times,* June 12, A27.

Dionne, E. J., Jr. 2005. Protect the rich: How Bush will 'reform' Social Security. *Commonweal,* March 11, 9.

Elderly Housing Coalition Committee on the Continuum of Care. 2000. Providing an affordable continuum of care for low-income residents of senior housing. Catholic Health Association. www.chausa.org/longterm/providing_er.asp.

Federal Interagency Forum on Aging-Related Statistics. 2000. Older Americans 2000: Key indicators of well-being. www.agingstats.gove/chartbook2000/Older Americans2000.pdf.

Harris, G. 2005. Gee, fixing welfare seemed like a snap. *New York Times,* June19, Week in Review, 3.

Hermalin, A. I., ed. 2002. *The Well-Being of the Elderly in Asia: A Four-Country Comparative Study.* Ann Arbor: University of Michigan Press.

Hollenbach, D. 2002. *The Common Good and Christian Ethics.* Cambridge, UK: Cambridge University Press.

Institute of Medicine. 1997. *Approaching Death: Improving Care at the End of Life.* Washington, DC: National Academy Press.

Joint International Research Group of the Institute for Bioethics, Maastricht, the Netherlands, and the Hastings Center, New York. 1994. What do we owe the elderly? Allocating social and health care resources. Special Supplement, *Hastings Center Report* 24(2):S1–12.

Makoni, S., and K. Stroeken, eds. 2002. *Ageing in Africa: Sociolinguistic and Anthropological Approaches.* Hamphshire, England: Ashgate.

New York Times. 2002. UN offers action plan for a world aging rapidly. *New York Times,* April 14, 4.

O'Brien, D. J., and T. A. Shannon, eds. 1992. *Catholic Social Thought: The Documentary Heritage.* Maryknoll, NY: Orbis Books.

President's Council on Bioethics. 2002. *Staff Background Paper: The Promise and the Challenge of Aging Research.* http://bioethics.gov/background/agingresearch .html.

President's Council on Bioethics. 2005. *Taking Care: Ethical Caregiving in Our Aging Society.* Washington, DC: President's Council on Bioethics.

Ter Meulen, R. 2002. Are there limits to solidarity with the elderly? In *Healthy Thoughts: European Perspectives on Health Care,* ed. R. K. Lie and P. T. Schotsmans. Pp. 329–36. Lueven and Paris: Peeters.

United Nations. 1999. *United Nations Principles for Older Persons.* www.un.org/ esa/socdev/iyop/iyoppop.htm.

United Nations. 2003. *World Population in 2300.* www.un.org/esa/population/ publications/longrange2/longrange2.htm.

U.S. Catholic Bishops. 1986. *Economic Justice for All.* www.osjspm.org/cst/eja .htm.

Williamson, J. B. 1997. Should women support the privatization of social security? *Challenge* 40(July–August):97–108.

CHAPTER 18

The Ethics of Aging

Question of Ends at the End of Life

LAURIE ZOLOTH, PH.D.

To stimulate thought on the issue of whether there is research that ought not to be pursued, I often pose the following scenario on my final exam.

You are sitting in a hotel in Boston, and a man comes up to you with a scheme. He is a scientist from a new technology company, and he has an idea that he claims will double the lifespan of the people who agree to be a part of the experiment. He cannot be sure, but he has done the basic science. It will involve dramatic manipulations of the natural world and serious environmental risk, but it will promote longer and healthier lives; it may lead to dramatic cures for diseases we have been unable to treat and that claim thousands of lives. We are not speaking of incremental changes or of small tinkering steps, but of a radical and *de novo* world of significant change. This change may alter the very meaning of aging and of the categories and meanings of the family: childhood, adolescence, and adulthood. It will allow for a considerable change in the reproductive process. Finally, because the technology required is vastly expensive, it will not be available to most people in the world, and the fundamental inequalities between poverty and wealth and between industrialized and developing regions will perhaps be deepened.

Do you approve this intervention? Why or why not? Should it be publicly funded?

Here is the part my students do not know: What is proposed is the separation of water for drinking from water used for waste. This single innovation dramatically changed the lifespan of the majority of U.S. citizens in the mid- to late nineteenth century. In Chicago, engineers reversed the flow of the Chicago River with huge pumps so that potable water was drawn from the deep center of the lake, far from the polluted shallows, and reversed the flow of the Illinois River so that the sewage of the city flowed backward toward the Mississippi. In Boston, in 1848, Lemuel Shattuck not only acted as the chief researcher for public health but also became its publicist, arguing for the rapid adaptation of the technology of water reclamation and sanitization at the state legislature. The Cochituate Water System was the best in the world, he argued. He also said, as most men of science thought at the time (and as most people would argue now), "We are at the most exciting time to be a scientist." In America, the mid-nineteenth century was a time of great growth in the elaborate structures for research: the founding of Johns Hopkins, the Rockefeller Institute, and the network of America's great research universities.

This shifting boundary between medical research and public health and politics was maintained throughout the Progressive Era as well. Well before antibiotics, even before screens and antiseptic technique, the struggle for public funding for two separate water systems, an idea that was called the Sanitation Movement, achieved dramatic changes in the single most central fact of human existence: that infants were largely perishable, and that child mortality exceeded 50 percent. That babies would largely die and that women too faced deadly risks in childbirth shaped the social, ethical, political, and cultural landscape. It was a fixity of life; it seemed to be merely the natural course of things, intuitively valid, that sorrow was linked to fecundity, for thus it had always been. Reflect just a moment on the actual human life of the creator of the Frankenstein myth (Shelley, 1967) that is invoked in every discussion of the specter of genetics: Mary Wollstonecraft Shelley, whose babies died in her arms over and over and whose own mother, Mary Wollstonecraft, died in childbirth. In the Progressive Era as in our time, science and technology were among the most vivid discourses of the polity. Feminist economist and Jewish scholar Jessica Peixotto, who understood that women's freedom was linked to the demand for women's and children's health, organized women in California for sanitation and pasteurization. The group of women who were Peixotto's students, newly graduated from the University of California at Berkeley, were only one of a dozen such groups across the country, in which bourgeois women, educated in the new university systems that admitted women, linked their energies with the trade union movement as it organized in the newly industrialized, largely immigrant urban workforce. Peixotto was thoughtful about her motivation (she was an economist but wrote that her inspiration was also from Jeremiah). How to release the poor from the great poverty of the Industrial Revolution? Her argument was that science, progress, and industry were not disasters, yet they were dangerous if uncoupled from social justice. Further, this research and technological expenditure— for clean water, for clean milk—was made against tremendous opposition. It was costly, risky, and subversive. Reformers such as Peixotto faced arguments from conservative religious communities that such reform (especially when focused on women's health) was a violation or negation of God's intention.

Water projects challenged the world and nature in precisely the same way big genomics or stem cell science challenges us here, asking about the goal and meaning of our ability to manipulate the facticity of the world, to bend it toward our purpose, to seek to undo a suffering that has defined us, to defy a finitude with our big technology-driven dreams. In reading the texts of opposition to pasteurization, one reads of the sanctity of the farm and of concerns about the quest for mastery over a divinely willed world.

Stem Cells and the Ethics of the Normative

Why begin a chapter on the ethics of stem cells and regenerative medicine with an historical account about the nineteenth century? I began with this thought experiment because we are asked to do, of course, a similar one in nearly all of the articles about stem cells that link stem cell research to aging. In the first reports of the discovery of stem cells in a 1999 *New York Times* magazine, a cover featured an elderly couple, absurdly gotten up in adolescent clothing, riding skateboards. The core problem was expressed in a caricature of the deepest fears of folklore, perhaps the fear of primate vulnerability: that the older generation would eat the young. When a reporter calls a bioethicist for a response to the ethical issues of stem cell research, the reporter is asking not only about the actual praxis of the activity (Is it ethical to destroy a human embryo? Is it ethical to make cells in culture? Have the gametes been obtained and the embryo derived justly and with proper attention to informed consent procedures?) but also if the future world that this may imply is a good one. The reporter's ethical questions are the same as those implied by my exam question: May we remake the world? What must we do about human suffering? How far will our reach for mastery take us?

It is important to understand that my students always react to the exam question in precisely the same way the audience at the conference at which this paper was presented reacted. They universally (and nearly completely) reject the project. Even if I give all the details about the project, as many as could be known prior to its working (for no testing was feasible), the idea is still rejected until I reveal that it is a sanitation project. It is the way we have come to understand technology itself, a response that philosopher Emmanuel Levinas (1987, 1996) describes as "paganism" in the face of technology. For ethics—at least for a theorist who is concerned about the theological importance of our judgments—is in large part about prophecy, about the guess of morality in the face of the unknown.

This idea—that genetic medicine and stem cell regenerative medicine should be opposed because they will create a posthuman future in which the present generation of elderly people will live forever—is actually seriously made with frequency. It is a staple of the list of arguments about the ethical issue. Yet it is an odd claim, and one that rests on several uninterrogated premises. In this essay I will look briefly at this issue and reflect on a few reasons why we might wish to reexplore the philosophical and theological principles on which it rests, just as we did when looking at the historical case story.

Public health has increased the average life expectancy by about seven hours every day for the past 100 years in the United States (Shuster, 2004). Against this steady and measurable change, we reflect on the entirely speculative nature of stem cell research, the exquisite difficulty of merely growing stable colonies of human cells, and we are led to ask, Why do stem cells carry the weight of our fears? After all, much of stem cell technology is observational, looking at how cells grow and differentiate and fail to grow; it is the basis of human disease. But why are we not worried about RNA research? It is hard to learn about telomerase capping, heterodimers, and conformational changes in protein structure, so we head off to the bottom of the slippery slope where we are experts: we know about cloned babies and Nazi atrocities.

However, the fear of living forever is most strongly connected with this research, and this anxiety is in contrast to the sort of concern that arose when other technologies were introduced (note that this objection was not raised to oppose cardiac medication or artificial hearts). But our concern around the ethics of aging itself is more fiercely located in this debate. In this debate, fundamental concerns about what it means to live within the normal limits of the species itself are raised and divide us.

Messianism and the Call for Vision

Why stem cells? Our attention is drawn to this research for two reasons. First, the researchers themselves tell us that this technology has fundamentally different applications than previous work in pharmaceutical development. Consider the statement by Robert Lanza in chapter 5 of this volume: "Stem cells raise the prospect of regenerating failing body parts and treating a wide range of disorders." This statement reminds us that the goal of the research is not to treat diseases but to cure them entirely. Lanza further reminds us that the potential for such cures could affect the entire course of history: "One day, millions of patients could benefit from this technology." Such claims are understood as in part scientific, in that they are the hope of the outcome of the basic research, and in part as a theological construct technically termed *premillennial.* In short, these are claims about how human agency will transform essential conditions of humanity in a progressive and determined way. It is the basis for our trust in and our funding of science, a trust medieval societies placed and funded in much the same spirit via the building of huge multiyear cathedral projects. We intend, via medical research, to build a better home for the place of humanity's best dreams.

Second, this type of research focuses our fears of the future as a future that is altered in a particular way because of the nature of stem cells. The work thus far—in the 2005–2006 period in which this paper is written—is nearly purely theoretical data, not therapy. Scientists are still learning signal by signal how one cell at a time differentiates. The goal is to understand, then, the potential of every human cell as understood on a sort of continuum. Here is the scientific sketch of the problem: One cell, the first cell made when the sperm and egg combine, then divides to create a set of blank, immortal cells, that first differentiate into two sorts—inner cell mass cells and trophoblastic cells (which will divide into the specialized cells of the placenta). The inner cell mass cells are the human embryonic cells, which will then differentiate to all and any cells. The cells are several things that are interesting to a moral philosopher, in the sense of their existence and their essence: They are immortal, like cancer cells, in that they have long and intact telomeres capping the ends of their DNA. Additionally, they are mutable, and perhaps fundamentally so. Theoretically, if scientists could understand the steps toward increasing differentiation, as they can do practically by the addition of growth factors that "push" the cell toward specific cell lineage fates, then they could also eventually learn how to reverse that process—to dedifferentiate adult cells, pushing them back to the embryonic state, one in which each cell is every/any cell. Hence the deconstructionist impulse of this science mirrors physics and literary theory, in which the "whole" is atomized, recombined, and meaning is made up of so many Lego parts. It is this sense of instability that unleashes the fears of creation *ex nihilo,* or of the possibilities of category shifts. Hence, even work on supposedly moral, safe, and stable "adult" or somatic cells may create this anxiety about the fundamentally destabilized world.

The Ethics of Aging in a World of Temporality

Why does this fear arise now? Why are we particularly concerned about the instability in the human lifespan now, and why now more than, as I noted, in the nineteenth century (when one would have far more reason to fear)? We are faced with a category error as we consider stem cell research from an ethical perspective—perhaps a category creep. We live in a complex historical moment with several convergent discussions about aging that merge into a peculiarly mean-spirited discourse about a world full of dangers.

Further, we have this discussion after a decade of fierce and failed discourse about health care reform, which began, in the 1980s, with salvos against the elderly by then–Colorado governor Richard Lamb and bioethics scholar Daniel Callahan, both of whom wondered aloud whether the use of health care services by the elderly at the end of life, prolonging lives of diminished quality, was a sort of expropriation of funding best used by children. The debate was a negotiation against a background of health care rationing that was based on QALYs ("quality of adjusted life years"). The rationing needed a fixed number of years for the theory to work *and* needed the idea that quality and quantity were coupled. In this debate the stakeholders had to negotiate a trade zone, and in this trade zone the currency of exchange was a certain sort of utility. This set the argument in place for our concern for the use of medicine for the old as inauthentic, or, in theological terms, a form of gluttony.

We also enter our debate in a time of anxiety about the future in general and the technological future in particular. The paganisms of a return to the world of nature seem elegiac, but with such yearning comes a certain fatalism about the suffering of the other. Against a fear of the future and a yearning to return to the past (a place in which the old stayed old), stem cells posit a world in which far more might be required. In other work (Zoloth, 2005) I have thought this belief to be a folie à deux, in that both promoters and detractors of stem cell research indulge in an eschatological rhetoric that is largely unknowable, as yet, largely fears or hopes. Many within religious communities, who embrace fundamentalisms in different traditions, link fear of science and fear of research to a deep unease about what the future will bring. They reflect a growing certainty that the end of days could well end in catastrophe. The fear of dystopia draws out a curious fundamentalism, linked with a fatalism about things modern and an attraction to the sweeter attachment of earlier times. Much of the literature of opposition to stem cell research draws deeply, if not exclusively, from such tropes.

As many have noted, we live in a world in which the traditions of comfort and healing are often at stake. Faced with the despair of a violent century and against an agonistic reality, the sacred canopy of faith traditions is shaken, the fear of death is unmediated—except by medicine. Thoughtful critics of medical technology (Hauerwas, 1987; Wheeler, 1999; Hall, 2005) suggest that technology drives us from a belief in an afterlife, toward a materialism driven by the need to fill aging with things, the gear and get-ups of late-stage capitalism. Medicine, for these critics, becomes merely one more set of possessions one can yearn for and purchase.

The current moral choices and reflections about the ethical meanings of aging are also framed against a complex baby-boomer fantasy of the self, one that has become more elaborate as we ourselves have aged. This generation of bioethics critics is temporary, located in a certain historical period, and geographically located in the lucky luxury of the developed world. Reflect, for a moment, on the cultural tropes and themes thus engendered: that our own parents cannot be trusted (don't trust anyone over 80); that they have terrible judgment, not real wisdom; that they are lost in a materialist delusion, a meaningless existence. Our tirades sound oddly familiar for children raised in the 1960s. One can reflect on the movies of the 1960s and 1970s (e.g., *The Graduate,* in which the protagonists clearly see their parents as "creepy," old and insensitive, and, yes, gluttonous).

This generation of scholars has historically led the way toward essential returns to the "natural" world, a popular movement as striking (and as different in direction) as the Progressives of the Sanitation Movement I cited at the beginning of this chapter. The progressive movements of the twentieth century called for spirituality, home birth, Earth Day, scorning the polyester leisure suits of the generation that preceded them. Beneath this politics lurked a quiet fear of our own predilection for selfish excess. Witness how this generation of students who became the scholars and critics of bioethics have clearly embraced the dying of our hair, the use of Viagra, a disturbing material gluttony reflecting our inability to set limits on consummations of resources. This last problem is held in tension with a widespread literature of a sense of scarcity—that this generation of humans will not have "enough of the world," that we will run out of space, air, water.

Our moral qualms about the poor and our frustration about the best way to help have led to an increasing call in public life for personal responsibility rather than the collective shouldering of burdens. In this we are pitted all against all, and the concern is raised: If my neighbor is kept alive, will there be less for me? Thus, a worry arises about intergenerational conflict whenever a new technology is proposed. Such fears were raised with organ transplants and are raised again in stem cell research.

It is correct to worry about this problem. (Why do we flee into childhood, run from the work of adult life, dye our hair to pretend we are 25-year-old graduate students?) It is right to write lyrical articles about the need to confront our terror of our loss, for it is indeed the case that our generation is driven by its fear of dying. Bioethics must critique new science with great care, however, for the danger is that we will provide the ideological basis for the erosion of the basic social contract: Social Secu-

rity, Medicaid, and unrelenting progress in public health research. Moral
panic against research has implications not only for the diseases that affect
elderly people but also for the diseases of children and for cancer, diabetes, and others.

The main argument opposing stem cell research because it will distort
the "essential" human condition is a lovely one from natural law: The
human lifespan has an order. Babies are born, they grow, they marry and
have more babies, and then they die. But let us carefully examine this argument. First, one must note that our sense of aging is a construct of the
twentieth century. There is nothing "natural" about that order. It is a *moral*
creation that we have politically struggled to achieve. It is achieved in the
developed world at the cost of the existence of a developed world with a
very different "natural" lifespan and fate, especially for women. Such a
"natural" lifespan is a victory of modernity itself. Biblical patriarchs were
rare, and grandmothers far rarer. (Rachel's postpartum grave at the side of
the road to Hebron was commonplace.) It was the struggle of the Progressive Era to understand that a world could be made (modernity in all its
complex beauty and terrifying power), but only if women's lives could be
unshackled from the tragic normalcy, the naturalness, of maternal and
infant mortality, from the world of Mary Shelley.

What Is Needed in the Debate?

Here are some ideas for a reply.

Asking the Correct Questions

We must first ask, What sort of a question is it to ask if we wish to live
forever, when in fact the science under discussion has not asked this question, nor is it interested in that quest? Scientists are thinking about the
alteration of illnesses that threaten and diminish cognition and mobility
at the end of life. Then why is this question so persistent? Is it, perhaps, a
way of medicalizing the deeper question: What sort of life is worth living?
As philosopher Samuel Flieshacker (2005) notes, it is this question that is
at the core of any reflection on the meaning of a moral life. Surely, he notes,
if ethics means anything at all, it means we can make a comment about
what makes a life worth living, what features and what criteria we are

seeking in making such a statement. Because we are bioethicists, we know that physical illness, suffering, loss of cognition, and loss of mobility or function are not human states that we seek out or valorize, however much we know that it is noble to face them with grace.

A Sober Grip

We need a sober grip on the long road to therapy (much less immortality) and a refusal to stop science for science fiction. As bioethicists, it is our duty to be honest and to be humble. We cannot know, and we cannot claim to know, about immortality. We ought to be honest about how far from any of these therapies the science researchers are at this time. If we insist that scientists avoid hype and false promises, we as bioethicists need to avoid hysteria and false threats.

A Theory of Justice

Are we entitled to good health? Are we Utilitarians? Equalitarians? Libertarians? Under what theory is it unjust to seek to treat or cure diseases if the side effect is that people will live longer? Why is that a credible argument? Would it be right if the intervention was available to all equally? Note that my favorite intervention, clean water, is absolutely *not* available to all equally. Should we have waited to act on the cleanliness of the water of Chicago until it was available to all? Should we have not developed antibiotics or monoclonal antibodies or insulin until these were available to all? Can science be funded only after the core distributive problems are adjusted? Of course not, we do not hold the standard of absolute equality of access for any other intervention.

Why is it wrong, empirically, to live longer (and why would it be "more wrong" to extend the human lifespan from 40 years to 60 years or more wrong to move from 80 to 96)? What is the nature of the wrong? Is it that my existence is unjust (the meaning of being old, the ontology)? Or is it that my relationship to production is unjust (my consumption)? If we were to turn to these questions, then we would see that the problem is what Kant (1998) would note is the lack of human flourishing. But that is a problem about the need for a meaningful life—for service and work. The problem with aging is the idea that retirement is a kind of endless recess.

This is a separate sort of discourse from considering how we take on the difficult problem of actual health care reform or address malarial swamps. It is a problem of what generations owe one another.

A Theory of Good and Evil

Rope Burns (Toole, 2000) is a collection of accounts of poor old men who find meaning in hard work, physical discipline, and durability. We admire these qualities because the heart of evil in modernity is that persons are disposable; one can be killed or used and then replaced. The stories, from which the movie adaptation *Million Dollar Baby* was made, are ones in which powerful older men make powerful moral choices. The oddity of the story is the utter refusal of race, class, or fate—or age—to be the determining factor in the moral choices faced. Limits are real, and oppression is real, but in these stories hard luck is merely where you start; it is not your fate. The suffering body is the limit of medicine. But the public did not think to stop polio vaccine because Roosevelt was a brave man, and his suffering noble, and we did not stop the development of streptomycin because Helen Keller was a noble force for good. The two sorts of discourse have little to do with one another.

If you believe limits are real (and good for humanity), then it would follow that it is logical to believe limits are possible. Slippery slopes and precautionary principles lack a rigorous theory about the difficult freedom of moral agents. Without agency, we can worry about consumption of the consumer, as if it were the demographic category we needed to consider as primary; we are fixed on this as a "real problem." The empirical evidence would seem to demonstrate that it is not that simple.

Is it troubling that antiwrinkle cream or Botox is widely used by TV stars and your ordinary colleague down the hall? I think it is odd, sad, but hardly the postmodern future, hardly the subject of such overwrought prose that sells our field. What your colleague needs is a good talking to—a friend to speak to him of his wrinkly beauty, a friend who will tell him that he is not existentially alone. But this need for theological interpretation is the task of the moral philosopher (even if this one thinks men should not wear pony tails). We cannot substitute a moral panic about the end of the human race in its difficult place.

Advice about How to Be Good

The bioethicist who is devoted to concern toward the human fate should be able to suggest a praxis of being that displays the good. Such was the legacy of Aristotle. Might I suggest that bioethicists who worry about the wasteful elderly urge the retired toward useful service work or toward a variant of an American Service Corps? (We could call this the Miami Virtue Project.) Such an idea is a good one, a moral one, and not a trivial matter. I am ready to cheerily suggest this idea to the very reformers who were eager to have welfare recipients be made to work. This idea of elderly service works in China, where the elderly care for the young. I can think of critically important uses for golf courses and spas—perfect places for camps for children, to name one. If we are worried about what could happen if the diseases of aging are in fact ever cured by stem cell research, we can insist that this time, bought by research and public funding for it, it is a sort of a debt, and that elderly people who are the recipients have a duty to give back to the society that offered it.

A Sense of History

Twenty years ago a small industry of critics grew up around this very question of medicine; it occurred long before genetics or stem cells. In 1987 Daniel Callahan made an argument that heart transplants and intensive care units would drastically change the human experience, and that this would distort medicine. I will end this short essay with a final thought question.

Callahan and others argued that we should ration medicine to the elderly because not doing so would change our society in rather radical ways. Have these fears come to pass in 20 years, one generation after the events that engendered them? It is a test question, so I will end by leaving it open.

REFERENCES

Callahan, D. 1987. *Setting Limits: Medical Goals in an Aging Society.* New York: Simon and Schuster.

Flieshacker, S. 2005. What do we mean when we say life is worth living? Northwestern University Philosophy Series, October.

Hall, A. L. 2005. Holy husbandmen: Virility and virtue in the "Keeping Fit" campaign of 1919. American Association of Religion, Panel on Childhood, November.

Hauerwas, S. 1987. *The Suffering Presence: Theological Reflections on Medicine, the Mentally Handicapped and the Church.* South Bend, IN: University of Notre Dame Press.

Kant, I. 1998. *Groundwork on the Metaphysics of Morals.* Cambridge, UK: Cambridge University Press.

Levinas, E. 1996. *Basic Philosophical Writings.* Bloomington: Indiana University Press.

Levinas, E. 1987. *Time and the Other.* Pittsburgh, PA: Duquesne University Press.

Shelley, M. 1967. *Frankenstein; or, the Modern Prometheus,* ed. M. K. Joseph. New York: Oxford University Press.

Shuster, E. 2004. Public health: Towards a disease-free life without end? The 131st Annual Meeting of the American Public Health Association, November 15–19, 2003. Published as abstract, 2004.

Toole, F. X. 2000. *Rope Burns: Stories from the Corner.* New York: Ecco Harper Collins.

Wheeler, S. 1999. Making babies? *Sojourner's* 28(3):14.

Zoloth, L. 2005. Under the fallen sky. European Union, Plenary Address, Bioethics and Humanities Seminar, Holland, April.

CHAPTER 19

A Lonely New World— or Me, Myself, and I

ROSEMARIE TONG, PH.D.

Before news broke of Dolly the cloned ewe, I was discussing limits on the right to procreate with one of my classes. I asked the students whether people have a right to engage in assisted reproduction—that is, to use the genetic material and/or gestational services of one or more individuals to help them bring a child into the world. The students had no major objections to infertile people using the gametes of sperm donors or egg donors to procreate, although some of the more thoughtful ones noted that most sperm and egg donors were not really donors but instead vendors who sold their genetic wares at market price. They also observed that it was far more risky to be an egg donor than a sperm donor; that it was not clear whether it was better for gamete donors to be anonymous or known to their recipients and offspring; and that something was deeply troubling about paying people increasingly high amounts of money for "special" gametes. Indeed, one or two students even had the courage to make a bona fide moral *judgment* and say that it was simply wrong to pay a woman $50,000 for her supposedly superior eggs (Leavens, 1999).

As I continued to probe the class, focusing on the subject of in-vitro fertilization in particular, students started to raise questions about the moral status of frozen pre-embryos—as many as 400,000 in the United States alone (Caruso, 2004). Were the individuals who produced them but no longer wanted them for their own procreative purposes free to discard them? To put them up for adoption? To earmark them for research, including stem cell research? What kind of custody claim might be made in the case of divorce or in a case in which the man but not the woman (or vice versa) wanted to procreate? Whose right prevails—the right of the person who does not want to procreate or the right of the person who does (Robertson, 1994)? Do men have the same right to "abort" their petri dish pre-embryos as women have to abort their in utero embryos? What about the pre-embryo? Does it have a right to be implanted in a woman's womb? If so, in whose? Should researchers develop artificial wombs for unwanted pre-embryos (Singer and Wells, 1995)?

Not surprisingly, questions about implanting pre-embryos prompted me to ask the class their views about surrogate mothers. Specifically, I asked the students who should get custody of the baby if the surrogate decided she wanted to keep it. Should it matter if the surrogate mother is gestating an embryo to which she has no genetic relationship as opposed to one for which she has provided the egg? Is the child to whom she gives birth half hers if she has provided the egg, but otherwise not? Are children property one owns? Some students thought that whether or not the surrogate mother provides the egg for the child, she is the real mother of the child on account of her gestational connection to it. They emphasized that the surrogate mother's sweat-equity, her nine-month task, gave her primary claim to the child. Other students vehemently disagreed. They insisted that the contracting couple's intention to rear the child trumped the surrogate mother's lived commitment to it throughout her pregnancy, a pregnancy she could end, after all. Mind over matter! Rational contract over emotional connection! A deal is a deal! Our surrogacy discussion reached fever pitch when one student proclaimed that surrogacy was no one's business except that of the parties who contracted to the arrangement, to which another student replied, "You mean it's okay for two men in civil union to hire a surrogate mother to carry a child to term for them?" "Why not?" protested one openly gay young man in the back row. "As long as they love the kid and bring it up properly, what's the harm?" (Annas, 2005).

Saving the even more contentious issues for last, I could not resist asking the class their opinions on reproductive cloning. I asked them how they would respond to me if I told them that I was going to take a year's sabbatical to have myself cloned in a special sort of way. Infertility experts would pump me full of drugs and hormones to jump-start my dormant menopausal womb. Then they would figure out some way to extract an egg from me. Next, they would enucleate that egg, replacing its DNA with the same DNA from one of my somatic cells so as to be able to replicate me in embryonic form. Finally, after two or three days, they would transfer my image and likeness back into my womb, confining me to bed, no doubt, for the rest of my pregnancy, which would probably end early with a sched-uled Caesarian section. The baby, my little identical twin, would then be put into my arms for me to rear as I saw fit, indeed in splendid isolation from anyone else's interference, if I so chose. "More power to you!" pro-claimed one of my students. A few minutes later another student said, "If you did that, I'd lose all respect for you. I'd pity your clone."

Only the limits of my imagination prevented me from sketching out to the class the kind of scenarios George Annas (2005) sketched in response to Rael, the cult leader who would clone all human beings as the first step toward our evolution into a new "posthuman" species. All of us would get to go around not only once but as many times as we wished, our minds "downloaded" each time into bodies especially cloned for us so that we could look and think the way we looked and thought at whatever stage of life we selected as our restart point. One student protested that he would not want to be a "Raelian" posthuman, that he had no desire to live as long as did, say, Methuselah, who made it to 429 years of age (Wade, 2001). I asked him why he did not want to live forever. He said he would probably get bored with life sooner or later. He hoped there was something more after life—something now, different, better. He couldn't be more specific.

Clearly, Raelian posthuman clones would not be human beings as we know them. Why, then, do some scientists want to create them? Does prog-ress really demand "speciescide"? If so, why do we get so upset when a nonhuman animal species nears the point of extinction? Why do we mobi-lize the troops to stop the impending tragedy? If we care about mountain lions and panda bears, should we not care about ourselves too?

Like George Annas and many others, I have serious concerns about "species- endangering techniques," including reproductive cloning and germ-line gene therapy. Calls for a ban on such procedures gain part of their strength from the ways in which some somatic cell gene therapy has caused considerable harm. They also gain momentum from the ways in which some animal reproductive cloning has not worked all that well (Annas, 2005).

Consider the tragic case of 18 year old Jesse Gelsinger (Stolberg, 1999). He underwent somatic gene therapy for the treatment of ornithine trans-carbamylase deficiency (OTC) at the University of Pennsylvania. OTC is a genetic disorder in which the enzyme necessary for the metabolism of the amino acid ornithine is lacking. The result of this condition is that the liver cannot remove the toxic breakdown product ammonia from the body. Jesse Gelsinger had a mild form of the disease, which could be controlled through diet and drugs. However, he and his family wanted him to be free of even these relatively small disease liabilities. A gene-altered virus meant to correct the enzyme deficiency triggered an adverse immune response that went out of control. Jesse Gelsinger died as a result. His family maintained that neither they nor Jesse had ever been informed about the full risks of the intervention. They also alleged that they were never told that despite 600 clinical trials, somatic cell gene therapy had never cured anyone of any disorder.

Although animal and reproductive-cloning experiments have been more successful than human somatic cell gene therapy experiments, they have not been *entirely* successful. Far from it. For example, in order to produce Dolly, the world-famous ewe to which I previously referred, Dr. Ian Wilmut and his colleagues used 277 enucleated eggs. Only 29 of these enucleated eggs developed to the blastocyst stage, and only one of these blastocysts (Dolly) was brought to term successfully (National Bioethics Advisory Commission, 1997). Moreover, reports indicate that because an adult somatic cell was used to clone Dolly, her body prematurely aged before she died in 2003. Unless efforts to clone sheep, cows, dogs, cats, monkeys, and other animals become much more safe and efficacious, there is every reason not to attempt human reproductive cloning. According to many experts, producing a single viable human clone would require scores of women to donate eggs and carry embryos, most of which would either not come to term or be born with major deformities. Annas, Andrews, and Isasi sum the situation up well when they refer to embryologist Stewart Newman's comment that it is unlikely "that a human created from the union of 'two damaged cells' (an enucleated egg and a nucleus removed from a somatic cell) could ever be healthy" (2002, 158).

But let us assume that the harm factors in reproductive cloning could be overcome. What, then, would be wrong with using reproductive and genetic technology for people to get the child of their dreams: a normal child, an enhanced child, or a child that looked just like them or someone they loved, admired, or desperately needed for one or more purposes? Similarly, what, then, would be wrong about using these technologies and others to enable one's clone to live on virtually forever, continually replicating its DNA?

Some people think that the answer to the questions just posed is that in most circumstances there would be nothing wrong with using technology for one's idiosyncratic procreative purposes. Lawyer John A. Robertson, for example, has vigorously defended parents' right to select their offspring's characteristics. As he sees it, parents have a specific right to select offspring characteristics that is linked to two more general rights: (1) the right *not to procreate* children, simply because of the more or less burdensome aspects (physical, psychological, and social) that are linked to bearing and rearing children; and (2) the right *to procreate* children with particular characteristics "because of the great importance to many individuals of having biologic offspring—personal meaning in one's life, connection with future generations, and the pleasures of child rearing" (Robertson, 1994, 152).

Robertson emphasizes, however, that like all rights, people's procreative rights are limited. They most likely protect "only actions designed to enable a couple to have normal, healthy offspring whom they intend to rear" (Robertson, 1994, 153). They are not likely to include actions intended to produce subnormal children, for example. Deliberately procreating "diminished" children would, in Robertson's estimation, probably "deviate too far from the experiences that make reproduction a valued experience" (166) to be protected by law. However, actions intended to produce supernormal children might, in his estimation, legitimately be viewed as part of "parental discretion in rearing offspring" (167).

To bolster his position on procreating enhanced children, Robinson notes that because society already encourages parents to improve their children *postnatally* through behavioral modifications, it should have no serious objection to parents improving their children *prenatally* through genetic modifications. In an attempt to bolster his point, Robertson enumerates some of the ways parents seek to change their already-born children. They send them to the best schools, give them music, art, and drama lessons, have their teeth straightened, and so on. Some parents go even farther than this. In the name of bettering their children, they submit their children to somewhat risky sex-alignment operations, elective cosmetic surgeries, growth-hormone treatments, Ritalin therapy, and multiple doses of Prozac. So long as preimplantation and prenatal genetic technologies are no more harmful than the postnatal measures just described, challenges Robertson, would not the most humane course of action be to let parents enhance their children before they are born? Why subject an already-born child to onerous beautification treatments and surgeries when one could instead genetically modify her in utero so that she could be born a natural beauty?

Implicit in Robertson's view is the idea that, ordinarily, enhancement of a fetus is beneficial but that diminishment of a fetus is harmful. Robertson's ideas about the nature of harm seem to be roughly equivalent to those of philosopher Norman Daniels (1986), who views as harmful any actions that decrease so-called species-typical functioning. If it is typical for the human species that its members be able to hear and see, then deliberately deafening or blinding a fetus would be harmful to the fetus. But the question remains whether, according to Daniels's view, actions that *increase* species-typical functioning are permissible. A close reading of Daniels's arguments suggests that positive "atypicalities" are not to be shunned in the same way that negative "atypicalities" are. So long as every member of the species can do what is typical for the species reasonably well, it matters not that some members of the species can do it exceptionally well. In fact, it might be good for the species if more of its members were "peak performers."

Given the reasonability of Robertson's and Daniels's positions on enhancement, it is difficult to identify what would, in the end, be wrong about enhancing one's progeny. Yet lawyer Dena Davis (1997) is able to provide some clues. She notes that because people are likely to disagree about what counts as an enhancement and what counts as a diminishment, deaf parents, wishing to ensure deaf children for themselves, may argue that the lifestyle in the deaf community is so good that they want to guarantee that their children will be able to be full participants in it (Davis, 1995). In essence, deaf parents might argue in the manner of Amish parents who defend their practice of limiting their children to an elementary school education on the grounds that further formal education interferes with the Amish system of home-based vocational training—that is, learning from your parents how to live a simple, "God-fearing, agrarian life."

Although most Americans believe it is parents' prerogative to shape the values and lives of their children, they also have reservations about Amish parents, for example, effectively confining their children to the Amish community before their children are mature enough to decide for themselves whether such a world suits them. Davis (1997, 565) notes that by depriving their children of the opportunity to secure a high school diploma, Amish parents come close to ensuring "that their children will remain housewives and agricultural laborers." Amish children who rebel against the Amish way of life for one reason or another will find themselves without the education they need to enter the highly competitive mainstream professional marketplace. In Davis's estimation, Amish parents wrong their children by substantially limiting their right to control the course of their own destinies. Davis then reasons that if Amish parents wrong their children by denying them educational opportunities, the lack of which will set them back considerably in the larger non-Amish community should they ever decide to enter it, deaf parents would even more egregiously wrong their children by using genetic therapies to permanently deprive them of their ability to hear. Davis comments, "Deliberately creating a child who will be forced irreversibly into the parents' notion of 'the good life' violates the Kantian principle of treating each person as an end in herself and never as a means only. All parenthood exists as a balance between fulfillment of parental hopes and values and the individual flowering of the actual child in his or her own direction . . . Parental practices which close exits virtually forever are insufficiently attentive to the child as an end in herself. By closing off the child's right to an open future, they deprive the child as an entity who exists to fulfill parental hopes and dreams, not his own" (569–70).

Although Davis's arguments are directed against the practice of what she regards as genetic *diminishment,* they give us an opportunity to ask whether genetic *enhancement* is necessarily better for children than not only genetic diminishment but also genetic *normalcy.* On the one hand, it seems that a genetically enhanced child would have a more open future than a normal child. For example, a person with exceptional intellectual capabilities will likely have the opportunity to pursue a much wider range of career options than a person with average intellectual capabilities. On the other hand, a genetically enhanced child might have a future more closed than a normal child if, for example, his parents enhanced his intellectual and rational capacities to such a degree that his physical and emotional capacities shriveled. There are historical precedents for such a concern. Using simply environmental means (education), philosopher John Stuart Mill's father, for example, overdeveloped his son's rational and philosophical talents and underdeveloped his son's emotional and poetic talents. As a result, Mill had a mental breakdown as a young adult.

Among the thinkers who worry that parents might wrong their children in their drive to improve them is bioethicist Glenn McGee. He claims that parents intent on enhancing their children are prone to sins such as "calculativeness," "being overbearing," "shortsightedness," and "hasty judgement" (McGee, 1997, 33). Parents might, for example, become so systematic and rational about improving their children that they deprive themselves and their children of a fully human parent-child relationship; or they might put so much faith in the power of genetics that they forget the strong role that environment plays in human development; or they might find themselves with a child who, despite all their interventions, still falls short of their expectations. Although such sins are not always "deadly," says McGee, they should nonetheless be avoided by an "intelligent" and "cautious" approach to using genetic technologies for the purpose of enhancement. Society should, he insists, "work toward developing protocols and therapies [for genetic enhancement] experimentally and gradually" (132).

Some of McGee's points are reinforced by philosopher Maggie Little. She worries that parents might be tempted to use genetic therapies as well as environmental therapies to shape their offspring to fit largely media-driven standards of human perfection, standards that often reflect and even idealize social values that remain regrettably racist, sexist, homophobic, and so on. For example, in a worst-case scenario, African-American parents might request lighter skin for their children, or parents of any race might request thin bodies and beautiful faces for their daughters. Little (1999) views such requests as morally disturbing because "the norms of appearance at issue are grounded in or get life from a broader system of attitudes and actions that are in fact unjust" (166). For African Americans to want their children to look more white than black is probably not "some aesthetic whimsical preference" (166), says Little. It is more likely a function of a racist history in which being black is devalued and being white is valorized. Similarly, for parents to want their daughters to look like fashion models or movie stars is probably not some aesthetic whimsical preference either, but more likely a function of a sexist history in which being an overweight plain woman is penalized economically and emotionally and being a thin attractive woman is rewarded. Rather than welcoming and encouraging diversity and change, many genetic enhancement activities would, in Little's estimation, aim instead for homogeneity and the further ossification of our unjust status quo.

Concerns about justice also occupy Maxwell Mehlman and Jeffrey Botkin in their analyses of genetic technologies, including those aimed at enhancement. As they see it, most of these technologies, but particularly enhancement therapies, will be accessible only to those parents who have expanded insurance coverage or who can afford to pay for them out of pocket. Mehlman and Botkin (1998) speculate that as a result of this situation society will be divided into two classes: a "genetic aristocracy" and a "genetic underclass." They comment that the former group "would be virtually free of inherited disorders, would receive powerful genetic therapies for acquired diseases, and would be engineered with superior physical and mental abilities" and that the latter group "would continue to suffer from genetic illnesses and would have to content itself with less effective, conventional medical treatments. Its members would be able to improve their mental and physical traits only through comparatively laborious traditional methods of self-improvement" (99).

As bad as the consequences of this divide would be for the individuals in the genetic underclass, Mehlman and Botkin think that the worst consequence of this state of affairs would be the destruction of democratic society. As they see it, a genetically stratified society would undermine social equality in three ways. First, it would increase *actual inequality* by enabling the genetic aristocracy to secure greater genetic health and talent than the genetic underclass. Second, it would erode the *belief in equality of opportunity* by enabling the genetic aristocracy to make themselves "the best and the brightest" and then to pass on their genetic advantages to succeeding generations. Finally, it would destroy the hope for *social mobility* in the genetic underclass, who would become increasingly resentful about their lot in life (102).

Mehlman and Botkin consider the possibility of banning genetic therapies or of asking health care professionals to voluntarily refuse to provide them, but they conclude that neither legal bans nor health care professionals' refusal to provide certain treatments will work in the long run. They stress that as soon as scientists develop genetic technologies that can eliminate, cure, or ameliorate serious genetic diseases and defects, the public will want not only technological products that can make them well but also technological products that can make them "better than well" (Elliott, 2003, 203). Thus, Mehlman and Botkin predict two inevitabilities. State authorities will permit a relatively free market in genetic services, and health care professionals will soften their practice guidelines to meet the public's demands for treatments and drugs that ward off sickness, degeneration, disintegration, aging, and even dying. But because only some people will be rich enough to secure expensive nontherapeutic as well as therapeutic genetic interventions, stress Mehlman and Botkin, there will be only two possible ways to save democracy: (1) creation of a system of genetic handicapping for the genetically nonenhanced; or (2) inauguration of a genetic lottery, open to all citizens for no cost, in which the prize is a complete package of genetic services. The latter option is the remedy Mehlman and Botkin favor on the grounds that the former option will not work because when something "important is at stake," like airline passengers' safety, people will not want "a pilot who had been hired over someone with better eyesight, or stamina, or quicker reflexes, simply in order to level the social playing field" (122).

Mehlman and Botkin's proposed solution to the problems that face us strikes me as a capitulation to people's whims and the goddess Fortuna's caprices. Although I agree with them that *bans* on reproductive and genetic technology will not work in the long run, I disagree with them that health care professionals will not be able to set limits on which reproductive and genetic services treatment they provide to patients. Mehlman and Botkin suggest that the main reason health care professionals will not be able to resist their patients' demands for enhanced offspring, including cloned offspring, is that there is no ultimate end, aim, or purpose of medicine with which to counter these demands. They imply that, in the end, medicine may simply be a set of techniques and tools used to attain whatever ends people have; and physicians and other health care professionals had best get used to the idea that they are nothing more than technicians who exist to please their patients (or is it customers?) (Kass, 1985). However, as I see it, it is not yet time to give up on the practice of medicine as we have known it. Caution suggests that physicians and other health care professionals should continue to (1) struggle to distinguish between health-related therapies, treatments, and drugs on the one hand and non-health-related ones on the other; and (2) provide to their patients only so many medical services as their health requires (Walters and Palmer, 1997).

This caution applies equally well to proposals to control aging. It is one thing to "compress morbidity" (Fries, 1980) so that the chronic diseases and disabilities that currently strike people around age 50 do not occur until age 90 or so, shortly before one is scheduled to die (Miller, 2002). However, it is quite another for medicine and science to wage war against death, working feverishly to find ways to indefinitely postpone aging and/ or to create posthumans (De Grey et al., 2002). Reading *Faust* (Goethe, 1998 translation) explains the difference. Human beings were meant to die.

Rather than claiming that health care professionals should provide non-health-related genetic therapies to people because they already provide them with elective cosmetic surgery and the like, perhaps we should re-consider the possibility that all such interventions fall outside the scope of the moral practice of medicine. Their aim is to make people happy and not simply healthy. Admittedly, just because members of the U.S. medical and scientific community refuse to provide non-health-related genetic therapies to people does not mean that some other group or persons will not. Rael, who wishes to download our brains into new bodies shortly be-fore our old bodies succumb to the "ravages" of aging, once again comes to mind.[1] So too does Dr. Seed, who wishes to clone himself in the meno-pausal womb of his wife, a woman in her sixties.[2] However, such rivals to the more noble traditions of medicine and science are not likely to succeed unless large numbers of health care professionals and scientists break ranks and join their company, a defection that even in these self-interested times I do not think is highly likely. There is still too much integrity in the medical and scientific professions for health care professionals and scientists to let people play gleefully with their destiny, let alone their progeny's.

For now I hope that we all ask ourselves why someone would want to have a perfect baby, indeed a cloned baby made in their own image and likeness or that of some valued third party (say, a deceased parent or child); or why someone would want to live forever, even if no new lives could be brought into the world. It strikes me that the answers to such questions might reflect an excessive need for control and power. Specifically, the quests for the perfect child and eternal life on earth are quests to get the world just the way one wants it for as long as one wants it, irrespective of the political, economic, and social havoc one causes. In my estimation, we should not spend our limited health care dollars on developing techniques to provide the wealthiest people in the world with the means to custom design their children or to achieve corporeal immortality in a series of cloned bodies. Instead, we should spend our money on providing high-quality universal health care coverage for everyone in the United States and on finding cures for the diseases that kill millions of children and infants annually throughout the world, thereby ending all too prematurely lives just as valuable as U.S. lives. Our task is to convince ourselves that we have a collective responsibility to create a just world in which all human beings can thrive. For if we create a world that is truly just, we may no longer feel a need either for perfect children or to live forever, so satisfied will we be with the idea of going around once, our imperfect children in tow, headed toward the end, the period, the death that will give our lives final meaning.

NOTES

1. See the Raelian Revolution website, www.rael.org.
2. See an article about Dr. Seed at http://news.bbc.co.uk/hi/english/sci/tech/newsid_166000/166216.stm.

REFERENCES

Annas, G. J. 2005. *American Bioethics: Crossing Human Rights and Health Law Boundaries.* New York: Oxford University Press.
Annas, G. J., L. B. Andrews, and R. M. Isasi. 2002. Protecting the endangered human: Toward an international treaty prohibiting cloning and inheritable alterations. *American Journal of Law and Medicine* 28:151–78.
Caruso, D. B. 2004. Clinics vary widely in embryo donation. *Charlotte Observer,* September 19, A10.
Daniels, N. 1986. *Just Health Care.* New York: Cambridge University Press.
Davis, D. 1997. Genetic dilemmas and the child's right to an open future. *Rutgers Law Journal* 28:549–92.
Davis, L. J. 1995. *Enforcing Normalcy: Disability, Deafness, and the Body.* New York: Verso.
De Grey, A. D. N. J., et al. 2002. Time to talk SENS: Critiquing the immutability of human aging. *Annals of the New York Academy of Science* 959:452–62.
Elliott, C. 2003. *Better Than Well: American Medicine Meets the American Dream.* New York: W. W. Norton.
Fries, J. F. 1980. Aging, natural death, and the compression of morbidity. *New England Journal of Medicine* 303:130–35.

Goethe, J. 1998. *Faust: Part One,* trans. David Luke. Oxford: Oxford University Press.

Kass, L. R. 1985. Perfect babies: Prenatal diagnosis and the equal right to life. In *Toward a More Natural Science: Biology and Human Affairs.* New York: Free Press.

Leavens, S. 1999. Students and professors react to egg donation ad. *Yale Daily News,* March 4. www.yaledailynews.com/article.asp?AID=1043.

Little, M. O. 1999. Cosmetic surgery, suspect norms, and the ethics of complicity. In *Enhancing Human Traits: Ethical and Social Implications,* ed. Erik Parens. Washington, DC: Georgetown University Press.

McGee, G. 1997. *The Perfect Child: A Pragmatic Approach to Genetics.* Lanham, MD: Rowman and Littlefield.

Mehlman, M. J., and J. Botkin. 1998. *Access to the Genome: The Challenge to Equality.* Washington, DC: Georgetown University Press.

Miller, R. 2002. Extending life: Scientific prospects and political obstacles. *Milbank Quarterly* 80:155–74.

National Bioethics Advisory Commission. 1997. *Cloning Human Beings: Report and Recommendations of the National Bioethics Advisory Commission.* Rockville, MD: The Commission.

Robertson, J. A. 1994. *Children of Choice: Freedom and the New Reproductive Technologies.* Princeton, NJ: Princeton University Press.

Singer, P., and D. Wells. 1985. *Making Babies: The New Science and Ethics of Conception.* New York: Charles Scribner's Sons.

Stolberg, S. G. 1999. The biotech death of Jesse Gelsinger. *New York Times Magazine,* November 28. www.nytimes.com/library/magazine/home/19991128mag-stolberg.html.

Wade, N. 2001. *Life Script: How the Human Genome Discoveries Will Transform Medicine and Enhance Your Health.* New York: Simon and Schuster.

Walters, L., and J. G. Palmer. 1997. *The Ethics of Human Gene Therapy.* New York: Oxford University Press.

INDEX

Page numbers in *italics* refer to figures and tables.